ALCOHOL
and COFFEE
USE *in the*
AGING

CRC SERIES IN MODERN NUTRITION
Edited by Ira Wolinsky and James F. Hickson, Jr.

Published Titles

Manganese in Health and Disease, Dorothy J. Klimis-Tavantzis

Nutrition and AIDS: Effects and Treatments, Ronald R. Watson

Nutrition Care for HIV-Positive Persons: A Manual for Individuals and Their Caregivers, Saroj M. Bahl and James F. Hickson, Jr.

Calcium and Phosphorus in Health and Disease, John J.B. Anderson and Sanford C. Garner

Edited by Ira Wolinsky

Published Titles

Handbook of Nutrition in the Aged, Ronald R. Watson

Practical Handbook of Nutrition in Clinical Practice, Donald F. Kirby and Stanley J. Dudrick

Handbook of Dairy Foods and Nutrition, Gregory D. Miller, Judith K. Jarvis, and Lois D. McBean

Advanced Nutrition: Macronutrients, Carolyn D. Berdanier

Childhood Nutrition, Fima Lifschitz

Nutrition and Health: Topics and Controversies, Felix Bronner

Nutrition and Cancer Prevention, Ronald R. Watson and Siraj I. Mufti

Nutritional Concerns of Women, Ira Wolinsky and Dorothy J. Klimis-Tavantzis

Nutrients and Gene Expression: Clinical Aspects, Carolyn D. Berdanier

Antioxidants and Disease Prevention, Harinda S. Garewal

Advanced Nutrition: Micronutrients, Carolyn D. Berdanier

Nutrition and Women's Cancers, Barbara Pence and Dale M. Dunn

Nutrients and Foods in AIDS, Ronald R. Watson

Nutrition: Chemistry and Biology, Second Edition, Julian E. Spallholz, L. Mallory Boylan, and Judy A. Driskell

Melatonin in the Promotion of Health, Ronald R. Watson

Nutritional and Environmental Influences on the Eye, Allen Taylor

Laboratory Tests for the Assessment of Nutritional Status, Second Edition, H.E. Sauberlich

Advanced Human Nutrition, Robert E.C. Wildman and Denis M. Medeiros

Handbook of Dairy Foods and Nutrition, Second Edition, Gregory D. Miller, Judith K. Jarvis, and Lois D. McBean

Nutrition in Space Flight and Weightlessness Models, Helen W. Lane and Dale A. Schoeller

Eating Disorders in Women and Children: Prevention, Stress Management, and Treatment, Jacalyn J. Robert-McComb

Childhood Obesity: Prevention and Treatment, Jana Pařízková and Andrew Hills

Alcohol and Substance Abuse in the Aging, Ronald R. Watson

Handbook of Nutrition and the Aged, Third Edition, Ronald R. Watson

Vegetables, Fruits, and Herbs in Health Promotion, Ronald R. Watson

Nutrition and AIDS, 2nd Edition, Ronald R. Watson

Forthcoming Titles

Nutritional Anemias, Usha Ramakrishnan

Advances in Isotope Methods for the Analysis of Trace Elements in Man, Malcolm Jackson and Nicola Lowe

Handbook of Nutrition for Vegetarians, Joan Sabate and Rosemary A. Ratzin-Tuner

Tryptophan: Biochemicals and Health Implications, Herschel Sidransky

Handbook of Nutraceuticals and Functional Foods, Robert E. C. Wildman

The Mediterranean Diet, Antonia L. Matalas, Antonios Zampelas, Vasilis Stavrinos, and Ira Wolinsky

Handbook of Nutraceuticals and Nutritional Supplements and Pharmaceuticals, Robert E. C. Wildman

Inulin and Oligofructose: Functional Food Ingredients, Marcel B. Roberfroid

Micronutrients and HIV Infection, Henrik Friis

Nutrition Gene Interactions in Health and Disease, Niama M. Moussa and Carolyn D. Berdanier

ALCOHOL
and COFFEE
USE *in the*
AGING

Edited by

Ronald R. Watson

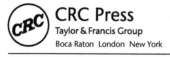

CRC Press
Taylor & Francis Group
Boca Raton London New York

CRC Press is an imprint of the
Taylor & Francis Group, an **informa** business

CRC Press
Taylor & Francis Group
6000 Broken Sound Parkway NW, Suite 300
Boca Raton, FL 33487-2742

First issued in paperback 2019

ISBN-13: 978-0-8493-2257-0 (hbk)
ISBN-13: 978-0-367-39805-7 (pbk)
Library of Congress Card Number 00-057196

Library of Congress Cataloging-in-Publication Data

Watson, Ronald R. (Ronald Ross)
    Alcohol and coffee use in the aging / Ronald R. Watson
            p. cm. — (CRC series in modern nutrition)
    ISBN 0-8493-2257-X
    1. Aged—Alcohol use. 2. Aged—Drug use. 3. Coffee—Health aspects. 4. Aged—Nutrition. I. Title. II. Modern nutrition (Boca Raton, Fla.)

RC564.5.A34 W38 2000
613.2—dc21   00-057196

**Visit the Taylor & Francis Web site at
http://www.taylorandfrancis.com**

**and the CRC Press Web site at
http://www.crcpress.com**

Series Preface for Modern Nutrition

The CRC Series in Modern Nutrition is dedicated to providing the widest possible coverage of topics in nutrition. Nutrition is an interdisciplinary, interprofessional field par excellence. It is noted by its broad range and diversity. We trust the titles and authorship in this series will reflect that range and diversity.

Published for a broad audience, the volumes in the CRC Series in Modern Nutrition are designed to explain, review, and explore present knowledge and recent trends, developments, and advances in nutrition. As such, they will appeal to professionals as well as to the educated layman. The format for the series will vary with the needs of the author and the topic, including, but not limited to, edited volumes, monographs, handbooks, and texts.

Ira Wolinsky, Ph.D.
University of Houston
Series Editor

Preface

As people become seniors, their physiology changes. Such biological changes make them more sensitive to alcohol and other abused drugs. Clearly, alcohol, tobacco smoke, and, to a lesser extent, caffeine in coffee, are addictive. It is difficult to discontinue use and abuse, and elderly people suffer from long-term and chronic exposure.

Alcohol use in elderly people is summarized, with an overview of the many types of physiological changes. Alcohol affects neurological and mental function and cognitive changes are accentuated by alcohol use, reducing the ability of elderly people to regulate or cease use. Mental function is damaged by both age and alcohol, which have some synergistic effects. Heart disease, the major killer of elderly people, is accentuated by alcohol use. Age, gender, and body composition influence the effects of alcohol in older people, affecting, as well, research outcomes and related conclusions. A detailed discussion of how alcohol affects the elderly population is presented for major types of health problems. The book includes an important description of how alcohol-using elderly people can be rehabilitated. A poorly defined synergism among alcohol abusers is the frequent association with tobacco smoking. These two agents are routinely used together, affect each others' intakes, and together promote the major causes of premature death in the elderly population. The role of alcohol abuse and tobacco smoking in elderly people is therefore carefully described and evaluated.

The most commonly ingested substance with addictive properties is coffee, via its caffeine. Caffeine is a major cause or contributing factor to insomnia in seniors. Its role and the mechanisms of action in the elderly population are described in detail. Coffee also has been associated with hypertension, cancer, and substantial health problems of many elderly people. The actions of caffeine and coffee that promote these conditions are defined.

The Editor

Ronald R. Watson, Ph.D., initiated the Specialized Alcohol Research Center at the University of Arizona College of Medicine and had directed the center for 6 years. Dr. Watson has edited 50 books, including 10 on alcohol abuse and 4 on other drugs of abuse. He has worked for several years on research for the U.S. Navy Alcohol and Substance Abuse Program.

Dr. Watson attended the University of Idaho but graduated from Brigham Young University in Provo, Utah with a degree in chemistry in 1966. He completed his Ph.D. degree in 1971 in biochemistry at Michigan State University. His postdoctoral schooling in nutrition and microbiology was completed at the Harvard School of Public Health and included a 2-year postdoctoral research experience in immunology. He was an assistant professor of immunology and did research at the University of Mississippi Medical Center in Jackson from 1973 to 1974. He was an assistant professor of microbiology and immunology at the Indiana University Medical School from 1974 to 1978 and an associate professor at Purdue University in the Department of Food and Nutrition from 1978 to 1982. In 1982, Dr. Watson joined the faculty at the University of Arizona in the Department of Family and Community Medicine. He is also a research professor in the University of Arizona's newly formed College of Public Health. He has published 450 research papers and review chapters and he also has directed a 20-year research project on aging, and a National Institute of Health grant on alcohol's effects on heart disease in AIDS.

Contributors

Åke Andreasson   Landvetter vårdcentral, Landvetter, Sweden

Marlene Oscar-Berman   Boston VA Medical Center and Division of Psychiatry, Boston University School of Medicine, Boston, Massachusetts

Becky T. Davies   Institute for Traffic Safety, Management and Research, Albany, New York

Michael J. Dunn   Department of Cardiothoracic Surgery, National Heart and Lung Institute, Imperial College School of Medicine, Heart Science Centre, Harefield Hospital, Harefield, Middlesex, United Kingdom

Robert Eggertsen   Department of Primary Health Care, Göteborg University, Mölnlycke vårdcentral, Mölnlycke, Sweden

Carlo La Vecchia   Istituto di Ricerche Farmacologiche "Mario Negri," and, Istituto di Statistica Medica e Biometria, Universita degli Studi di Milan, Milan, Italy

Patrick McNamara   Division of Psychiatry, Boston University School of Medicine, Boston, Massachusetts

John Dickson Mulinga   EMI Unit, Altham Meadows, Morecambe, United Kingdom

Vinood B. Patel   Department of Clinical Biochemistry, Guy's, King's and St. Thomas Medical School, King's College London, London, United Kingdom

Victor R. Preedy   Departments of Clinical Biochemistry and Nutrition and Dietetics, King's College London, London, United Kingdom

Peter J. Richardson   Department of Cardiology, King's College Hospital, London, United Kingdom

Jerry Seymour   Michael Carlisle Centre, Netheredge Hospital, Sheffield, United Kingdom

Alessandra Tavani   Istituto di Ricerche Farmacologiche "Mario Negri," Milan, Italy

Ronald R. Watson   College of Public Health, University of Arizona, Tucson, Arizona

John P. Wattis   Leeds Community and Mental Health Services, Park Hospital, Leeds, England

Simon Worrall   Alcohol Research Unit, Department of Biochemistry, The University of Queensland, Brisbane, Queensland, Australia

Hilary A. Wynne   Department of Elderly Services, Newcastle upon Tyne, United Kingdom

Jin Zhang   College of Public Health, University of Arizona, Tucson, Arizona

Contents

1

Alcohol Abuse in Elderly People: Overview and Summary

John P. Wattis and Jerry Seymour

CONTENTS

Introduction

A review at the beginning of the 1990s examined some issues concerning the epidemiology and diagnosis of alcohol abuse in old age.[1] It concluded that, although alcohol problems in this age group were still often hidden and poorly understood, they:

- Constituted a public health problem of moderate proportion
- Would probably increase in coming generations
- Might be of late onset as well as include some long-term abusers
- Were often not properly identified and present screening and diagnostic methods were not adequately validated for elderly people

Despite an increase in publications in this area, these conclusions remain broadly true. This is illustrated by an attempt to validate the well-known "CAGE" questionnaire in older primary care patients.[2] The CAGE detected fewer than half of heavy or binge drinkers. Asking additional questions on quantity and frequency of drinking increased the number of problem drinkers detected. The natural history of alcohol abuse in mid- to late life is now better understood, at least in selected populations.[3]

Epidemiology

Drinking habits, alcohol abuse, and alcohol dependence should be considered separately. Alcohol abuse is defined broadly as sufficient alcohol intake to cause physical, psychiatric, or social harm. The Diagnostic and Statistical Manual IV Edition (DSM-IV) defines abuse as a maladaptive pattern of substance use leading to clinically significant impairment or distress as manifested by one or more of four markers:

1. Failure to fulfill major role obligations
2. Recurrent use in physically hazardous situations
3. Substance-related legal problems
4. Continued use despite persistent or recurrent social or interpersonal problems[4]

Alcohol dependence is a particularly severe form of abuse characterized by development of unpleasant (and sometimes life-threatening) withdrawal symptoms 12 hours or so after reduction of intake following prolonged heavy drinking. The International Classification of Diseases 10th Edition (ICD-10[5]), uses the term *harmful use* rather than abuse and gives the following useful diagnostic guidelines for dependence syndrome:

- A strong desire or compulsion to take the substance
- Difficulties in controlling consumption

- A physiological withdrawal state
- Evidence of tolerance
- Progressive neglect of alternative pleasures or interests
- Persistence despite clear evidence of harmful consequences

Abuse (harmful use) is much more common than dependence, but problems exist in defining the borderline between ordinary "social" drinking and abuse, especially in elderly people. In Britain, the Royal Colleges of Physicians and Psychiatrists[6] suggested 21 units (a unit is defined as being roughly equal to a single shot) of alcohol per week as the upper "safe" limit for men and 14 units for women, but this makes no allowance for the changes in alcohol metabolism and distribution that occur with aging. Problems also exist in applying the same survey methods to younger and older groups of people. Older people may be less accustomed to surveys than younger people and may be more reluctant to disclose details of what they regard as "personal" matters, such as drinking behavior. It has even been suggested that they might fear that a "bad report" might lead to curtailment of social security benefits.[7] In addition, a higher proportion of elderly heavy drinkers might have memory deficits, rendering their self-report unreliable. The type of beverage consumed has been shown to affect social consequences[8] of alcohol abuse, but there is no specific work linking this to aging.

Surveys provide only a cross-sectional picture of drinking habits and use different definitions of light and heavy drinking. They are unable to distinguish among changing drinking habits as individuals grow older, period effects (relating to general social trends), and cohort effects between generations. Recent work has suggested that all these factors play a part in determining differences between older and younger people's drinking habits.[9] Surveys also do not allow for the different effects of social and financial pressures on different age groups. Knupfer and Room[10] asked people about past as well as present drinking habits. They found that there were slightly more older than younger people who currently abstained, having been alcohol drinkers in the past, and that lifelong abstention was much more common in the older age group. The older age group were in their teens and 20s during the era of prohibition in the U.S. and may therefore never have acquired the habit of drinking alcohol. Two surveys conducted in the Camberwell area in London in 1965 and 1974 illustrated changes in drinking patterns.[11] They showed an increase of nearly 50% in total alcohol consumption across the age groups with a nearly 100% increase in the over-55-year-old group. This, again, could be explained partly as a period effect, partly as a cohort effect, and partly as a result of different social and financial pressures on the different age groups. More recently, a study in New Zealand[12] of a community-based sample of people over 70 found that nearly a third of women and nearly two thirds of men reported that they drank less alcohol than they had in middle age, while 7% of men and 11% of women said they drank more.

With all the reservations above, it is, nonetheless, possible to give some over-all figures for "problem" and "heavy" drinkers. An editorial in the *British Medical Journal* estimated that 5 to 12% of men and 1 to 2% of women in their 60s were problem drinkers and that rates were higher in those attending hospital outpatient clinics.[13] In the U.S. between 2 and 4% of the elderly population met DSM-III criteria for alcohol abuse and up to 10% were heavy or problem drinkers.[14] A more recent large-scale U.S. survey in Erie County, NY[15] gave an overall self-reported prevalence of heavy drinking in the over 60 group as 6% with associations between heavy drinking and being male, having suburban residency, lower social status, and current smoking. Degree of health orientation was negatively associated with heavy drinking, but age (within the elderly population) and active lifestyle did not contribute to the model in this study. The authors suggested that health orientation offered the greatest opportunity to address heavy drinking among the elderly population.

There is considerable variation in specific subgroups of the elderly population. In patients presenting to primary care services in the U.S.,[2] 15% of male and 12% of female patients drank more than the limits suggested by the National Institute of Alcohol Abuse and Alcoholism (14 units per week for men and 7 units per week for women). Taking a more obviously harmful level of 21 units for both sexes, 9% of men and 2% of women drank over the weekly limits. The CAGE screening tool was not particularly useful in this population. The excess of male over female heavy drinkers is noteworthy in all studies. A recent review[16] also concluded that current tests were not very useful in screening for hazardous alcohol use in elderly people and highlighted the need for research on the consequences of lower levels of consumption on health and into the detection of alcohol problems in old age. In Australia, the prevalence of problem drinking in hospital inpatients was high. Problems with alcohol abuse were found in 99 of 640 elderly patients screened and only a third of these were identified by medical staff.[17] In retirement communities in the U.S., a recent study[18] has confirmed that many elderly people are regular drinkers but questioned the suggestion that these communities have a particularly high prevalence of heavy drinking. Similarly, despite some anecdotes, alcohol consumption in older urban American Indians does not differ from that in the general elderly population.[19] However, ethnic factors may be important as a Brazilian study found trends to increased rates of alcoholism in blacks and mulattos,[20] although this may have been confounded by socioeconomic variables. One review[21] closes with a plea for further research, especially among ethnic minority and homeless older people.

Four older U.K. studies throw further light on the complexities of drinking behavior in older adults and their ascertainment. Edwards et al.[22] found that alcohol abuse was not known to agencies in as many as eight of nine cases. They also found that, whereas rates for men were much higher than for women, the female rates peaked later, after age 70 rather than age 50. In Newcastle,[23] only 16% of the people over 60 were abstainers and men consumed an average of nearly 23 units per week, women 11 units per week, with the people under 75 consuming twice as much as those over 75.[23] In Islington and Brent, a study confined to those over 75 found nearly 50% of the men and over 75% of the women reported abstinence and only 4% of men and 3% of women were consuming over 21 and 14 units per week, respectively.[24] In Liverpool, a much larger study found a point prevalence for alcohol dependence of only 0.3%, but 6.1% of men and 2.4% of women admitted to regularly exceeding Royal College guidelines.[25]

On the evidence so far adduced we can conclude:

1. Cultural variation in drinking habits is prevalent among elderly people, even within a single country, with age, cohort, and period effects probably all playing a part.

2. For men, alcohol intake probably peaks in the fifth decade but remains relatively high in the 65 to 74 age range, falling off thereafter.

3. For women the age-specific rate may not vary so much, but may continue to rise into extreme old age at least in some cultures, although it is still low compared with men.

4. Men are more likely to be regular drinkers in all age ranges.

5. Women who do drink regularly are as likely as men to drink excessively.

6. Up to 10% of the U.S. elderly population are "heavy" or problem drinkers although only 2 to 4% meet DSM-III criteria for alcohol abuse.

7. In the U.S. and U.K. men are up to five times more likely to be problem drinkers than are women.

Etiology and Subclassification of Alcohol Abuse

Genetic factors play a part in the etiology of alcohol abuse, although they are probably of lesser importance with increasing age of onset. A recent twin study with a large number of identical and fraternal twin pairs ages 50 to 96 estimated the genetic variance at 38.5% and the variance for shared environmental influence at 15.5%.[26] The "medical, genetic, illness" model has been criticized on the grounds that it takes away responsibility from the individual,[27] and alternative, complementary psychological models have been proposed.[28] In old age, two distinct subtypes of alcohol abuse were identified, depending on age of onset.[29] This was confirmed by the work of Atkinson and colleagues[1,30] in the U.S. and Hauser and Rybakowski[31] in Poland. One review estimates that about a third to a half of elderly alcoholic individuals experience onset of problem drinking in mid- to late life.[32] Those who start abusing alcohol while younger and survive into old age are more likely to have a family history of alcohol abuse, to have a history of smoking, and to have a greater alcohol intake. By contrast, a late-onset group more often has an obvious precipitant for the onset of heavy drinking, a milder, more-circumscribed drinking problem, a more stable premorbid personality, and a better prognosis with appropriate treatment. Women may be relatively overrepresented in the late-onset group, at least in certain settings.

Physiology of Alcohol in Elderly People

Table 1.1 demonstrates the wide range of alcohol content in different drinks. The rate of alcohol absorption depends on several factors. The higher the concentration of alcohol, the more rapidly it is absorbed; carbon dioxide accelerates and sweetness slow absorption. Food in the stomach slows absorption markedly. There are no known age differences in absorption. After absorption, alcohol is distributed throughout the body and differences in lean body mass and total body water probably result in higher concentrations of alcohol per unit when consumed by an elderly person.[33] Most alcohol is metabolized in the liver and only 2 to 5% is eliminated unchanged via the kidneys and lungs. Chronic, heavy consumption of alcohol initially induces liver enzymes so that metabolism is accelerated and there is probably a synergistic effect with smoking. When liver damage supervenes, decreased metabolic capacity may be one of the factors related to a change in tolerance. Although ethanol is the main drug in alcoholic beverages, they also contain various amounts of different congeners that impart characteristic flavors and may also have pharmacological effects.

TABLE 1.1

Alcohol Content of Different Beverages

Group	Examples	Alcohol (%)
Beers	Lager	3–6
	Ales	3–6
	Stout	4–8
Table wines	Red, white, and rose (still)	8–14
	Champagne (sparkling)	12
Distilled spirits	Brandy	40
	Whisky	37–40
	Rum	40
	Gin	37–40
	Vodka	57.5
Liqueurs		20–55

Source: Royal College of Psychiatrists.

General Effects

High concentrations of alcohol damage human tissue. Drinks of 40% concentration or more may cause inflammation of the gastric mucosa, and lower concentrations may cause damage in predisposed patients by stimulating gastric secretions. Once in the bloodstream, alcohol causes a small, transient increase in heart rate and a dilatation of cutaneous blood vessels. This can lead to hypothermia in elderly people, especially as high levels of alcohol can also impair the temperature-regulating function of the brain. Very high concentrations of alcohol can cause respiratory and circulatory failure and death.

Effects on the Central Nervous System

In low doses, alcohol produces a subjective sense of well-being and alertness. This may be related to different effects on different neurotransmitter systems or to biphasic or even triphasic effects on individual systems. The GABA-benzodiazepine and dopaminergic systems are particularly involved. At the psychological level, these effects may be attributed to disinhibition. Table 1.2 summarizes the progressive effects on brain function as blood alcohol level rises. The aging brain may react differently to alcohol. For example, Helderman et al.[34] have shown that, whereas alcohol simply suppresses the secretion of antidiuretic hormone in younger people, in older people the hormone is initially suppressed but then rebounds to twice the basal level. This change in response may reflect other differences in neurohormonal response to alcohol in elderly people.

TABLE 1.2

Effects of Increasing Levels of Blood Alcohol

Blood Alcohol Level (Approx. mg%)	Effects
30	Driving skill affected
50	Disinhibition and increased reaction time
80	Risks of road accidents doubled
100	Clumsiness and emotional lability
200	Clear impairment of movement and emotion
300	Gross intoxication
500–800	Death

Drug Interactions

Adverse drug reactions occur more commonly in elderly people in the community and in the hospital. They are more severe than in younger people and result in higher rates of hospital admissions. Age is only rarely a primary risk factor for adverse drug reactions (for example, increased central sensitivity to the benzodiazepines). In most cases, the risk is secondary to multiple pathology, individual variation, or polypharmacy.[35] In a U.K. general-practice study, 87% of people aged 75 or over were having regular drug treatment and 44% were believed to be taking three or more drugs regularly.[36] The risk of interactions between prescribed drugs and between prescribed drugs and nonprescribed drugs (including alcohol) rises exponentially with the number of drugs taken. The acute effect of alcohol is generally to inhibit drug metabolism so that action is prolonged. Sustained heavy drinking first leads to enzyme induction, which may speed metabolism; then, as liver damage supervenes, metabolism is impaired. Aging itself produces changes in drug metabolism. Absorption is unaltered but reduced body weight and body water, combined with a relative increase in body fat and a lower concentration of plasma albumin produce complicated effects on distribution. Oxidation of some drugs (e.g., chlormethiazole) is decreased whereas others (e.g., diazepam) appear to be oxidized as readily as in younger people.[36] Renal elimination of some drugs is increased. The final result in an elderly individual taking alcohol and other drugs depends on complicated interactions, but the potential for harm is clear. Alcohol may also interfere with patient compliance with medication either through forgetfulness or through deliberate omission of medication for fear of interactions.

Natural History and Outcome of Alcohol Abuse in Old Age

The average alcohol intake in men is greater than in women at all ages. However, in old age the differences narrow somewhat due to a relative decline in male drinking. Some alcohol abusers die young, but half to two thirds of elderly alcohol abusers are "survivors" who have been abusing alcohol since early adulthood. The other third to a half have only started to abuse alcohol in late life. The first group tends to have more alcohol-related problems and the second group, who may start to drink more heavily following "loss" events, generally have less severe problems and may be more amenable to help if social networks can be reconstructed. Women are probably overrepresented in the late-onset group. Male late-onset alcohol abusers more closely resemble social drinkers,[37] and the same is probably true of late-onset female abusers. Over all age groups, women probably start to abuse alcohol a few years after men and first experience alcohol-related problems after a greater interval, although once problems occur women are more likely to present for treatment.[3] Abusing alcohol at any age increases morbidity and mortality, but the effects are more marked in older people who have fewer "functional reserves" to withstand the toxic effects of ethanol.

Damage

General

Mellstrom and colleagues[38] examined a sample of 468 70-year-old men and reexamined 342 of them five years later together with a cohort comparison group of 489 70-year-olds. About 10% met their criteria for "recidivism" (registration twice or more with the temperance board for previous alcohol abuse or large-scale alcohol consumption). The morbidity for diabetes, chronic bronchitis (corrected for cigarette consumption), the consumption of care, and mortality rate were higher in this alcohol-abusing group. They also had a reduction in the following indices: cognitive tests, muscle strength, "gonadal function" (measured by plasma lecithin:isolecithin ratio), pulmonary function, visual acuity, walking ability and skeletal density. Significant differences were found in blood glucose, plasma free fatty acids, and serum aspartate amino transferase activity, which were all higher in the recidivists. Unfortunately, the recidivists, while similar to the control group in nearly all demographic variables, did have a shorter time in education and a lower income than the nonrecidivists, so that it is possible that some of the differences were due to factors other than alcohol consumption. Current consumption is not the only issue. The Liverpool longitudinal study[25] has shown that men with a history of heavy drinking for five years or more at any time in their lives have a fivefold greater risk of suffering psychiatric disorder, mostly dementia or depression, in old age compared with those who have never been long-term heavy drinkers.

Medical Complications

All systems of the body may be affected by alcohol abuse. A direct causal link between alcohol abuse and pathology is clear in some conditions such as cirrhosis of the liver. In other cases the link may be more indirect; for example, alcohol may cause hypertension, but in any individual other factors such as heredity, obesity, smoking, diet, and lack of exercise may also contribute. Smoking is a particular confounding factor because many people who abuse alcohol also smoke heavily and both smoking and alcohol abuse are implicated in several conditions such as peptic ulcer and ischemic heart disease.

The reader is referred to a series of reviews dealing with trauma,[39] liver disease,[40] gastrointestinal bleeding,[41] infections,[42] cardiac disease,[43] and electrolyte abnormalities[44] in relation to alcohol. A separate review considered alcohol and the pancreas.[45]

Alcohol abuse and poor nutrition commonly coexist in elderly people for several reasons.[46] People who drink alcohol excessively may neglect their diet or may suffer reduced appetite as a result of alcoholic gastritis or peptic ulceration. Malabsorption may occur due to gastritis, pancreatitis, or diarrhea. Alcohol metabolism demands additional vitamins through enzyme induction and increased requirements of cofactors for oxidative metabolism. Ethanol itself may have a direct toxic effect on cell metabolism. Alcohol abuse can therefore lead to severe vitamin deficiencies (most notably C and B group) by several routes.

Alcohol abuse impairs the immune system, resulting in increased susceptibility to infection, including tuberculosis. The probable mechanisms include an effect on T cells and cell-mediated immunity[47] and an indirect effect through liver damage.[48] Alcohol is a risk factor for gastrointestinal malignancies, including large bowel cancer.[49] The mechanism probably relates to repeated damage and regeneration. Alcohol may also contribute to other cancers including breast cancer,[50,51] probably by interfering with immune surveillance. Liver cirrhosis is a disease that predominantly affects heavy drinkers in late middle age or those who are characterized as "young elderly" (i.e., aged 65 to 74). A study from the U.S.[52] showed the highest age-specific incidence of cirrhosis in men living in urban areas was in the seventh decade, while a French study[53] found that one fifth of patients with alcoholic liver disease were over 60 at presentation. Prognosis is also age related; the one-year mortality in those presenting over 60 was 50%, compared with 7% in younger patients.[54] Cardiovascular problems are also associated with alcohol abuse, with a higher risk of mortality from hypertension, hemorrhagic stroke, and cardiomyopathy.[55] It remains unclear whether or not a small amount of alcohol has a cardioprotective effect, as many factors other than alcohol intake probably affect the "J-shaped" mortality curve.[56] Chronic abuse and malnutrition can cause a painful, subacute sensorimotor peripheral neuropathy. This is symmetrical and usually most pronounced in the legs. A burning sensation in the soles of the feet, distal muscle weakness, and tenderness are the most common features.[57]

Neuropsychiatric Complications

Neuropsychiatric complications of alcohol abuse are common.[28,58] They can be divided into three phases: (1) acute intoxication; (2) withdrawal phenomena; and (3) chronic brain damage.

Acute intoxication — Acute intoxication is a rare presentation in old age. The differential diagnosis of an elderly person presenting in coma and smelling of alcohol includes a subdural hematoma and overdose.[59] *Pathological drunkenness*, when someone behaves out of character in a sexually disinhibited or violent way, after a relatively small amount of alcohol, may indicate subclinical brain damage (e.g., incipient Alzheimer's disease). *Wernicke's encephalopathy*[60] is characterized by ophthalmoplegia, ataxia, and delirium. It is probably due to acute thiamine (vitamin B1) deficiency and is a medical emergency which, if not treated promptly, can lead to the permanent deficit of Korsakoff psychosis.

Withdrawal phenomena — The withdrawal phenomena range in severity from tremulousness accompanied by irritability, anorexia, depressed mood, and insomnia to *delirium tremens* with extreme agitation, autonomic overactivity, visual hallucinations, confusion, and paranoid ideation. Delirium tremens can be a life-threatening condition although prompt diagnosis and supportive medical management have reduced the mortality rate of 15% suggested in some older texts, with one recent publication finding no mortality associated with a series of 539 episodes of general hospital withdrawal (all ages).[61]

Chronic brain damage — Chronic brain damage takes several forms. Alcoholic dementia is the clinical picture of gradual personality change and deteriorating memory. Joyce[62] suggests that all may be seen as variants of the Wernicke–Korsakoff syndrome and argues strongly for rigorous attention to the nutritional state of all alcoholics. Excessive drinking is often denied, sometimes with the collusion of family members.[63] The effect may be euphoric, fatuous, depressed, or labile. There may be greater impairment of judgment and social and sexual disinhibition than is normal in Alzheimer's disease and vascular dementia, although in practice there is considerable clinical overlap.

CT scan appearances in alcoholic dementia are similar to Alzheimer's disease. There is a decrease in brain size, widening of sulci, and enlargement of the ventricles. However, ventricular enlargement may resolve on abstention[64] in alcoholic dementia, probably as a result of neuronal plasticity and of rehydration.[65] There is some suggestion that women are more likely to show CT changes than men and that these may be more readily reversible.[66,67]

Pathologically, neuronal loss is particularly marked in the neocortex, basal ganglia, hippocampus, and reticular activating system. Impairment of cognition and psychomotor skills can be demonstrated on neuropsychological testing.[68,69]

The differential diagnosis between alcoholic and other forms of dementia in old age is particularly difficult, and it is likely that the contribution of alcohol to dementia is underestimated, especially since there are probably many cases of mixed pathology. Theoretically, one might expect an increased rate of vascular dementia in alcohol abusers in view of the known associations between alcohol and hypertension.[70] The complicated diagnostic picture is illustrated by results produced from different surveys. Of 35 elderly alcoholic individuals presenting to psychiatric, psychogeriatric, and alcoholism services in a Scottish survey, 17 had alcoholism, 1 had Korsakoff psychosis, and 6 had alcoholism with organic or senile dementia.[71] Some 17% of "indigent" elderly people admitted to a county psychiatric screening ward in the U.S. were diagnosed as alcoholic, while a further 27% had alcoholism with an associated chronic brain syndrome.[72] In neither study were the authors able to differentiate consistently between dementia due to alcohol and that due to other causes. A recent review examines this complex subject in some detail[73] and suggests that "heavy alcohol use" may be a contributing factor in 21 to 24% of cases of dementia.

Another form of chronic brain damage is *Korsakoff psychosis* which commonly follows Wernicke's encephalopathy. Even with treatment, only 20% of those with Wernicke's encephalopathy recover fully and 55% are left with unequivocal Korsakoff psychosis.[60] This is characterized by apathy, the inability to learn or form new memories, loss of insight, and confabulation. Confabulation is not diagnostic, as it also occurs in senile dementia.[74] Some patients appear otherwise mentally intact, although there is often subtle evidence of more widespread cognitive deficits and many patients have coexistent alcoholic dementia. CT scan shows particularly marked frontal brain shrinkage in patients with Korsakoff psychosis compared with other chronic alcohol abusers and normal controls.[75] With time, up to 25% of patients with Korsakoff psychosis make a full recovery and 50% a partial recovery,[76] although one study showed improvement in only 14% of patients over a five-year period.[77]

Alcoholic cerebellar deterioration produces progressive ataxia, dysarthria, and gaze-evoked nystagmus.[78] This condition, which is probably due to the direct toxic effects of very high alcohol levels, is found in binge drinkers and "skid-row" populations. It is rare to see onset in old age, although sometimes patients suffering from this complication survive into late life. The clinical picture is similar to that of subacute cerebellar degeneration due to carcinoma of the bronchus and a chest X-ray is always indicated. At autopsy, one third of chronic alcohol abusers had macroscopic cerebellar atrophy,[79] suggesting that this problem may be more widespread than is recognized clinically.

Alcoholic hallucinosis is characterized by persistent auditory hallucinations, usually derogatory or hostile in nature. It is rare in old age and occurs in the context of prolonged heavy drinking.[28]

Morbid jealousy secondary to alcohol abuse predominantly affects men and is characterized by morbid delusions that the spouse or partner is being sexually unfaithful.[28] This kind of delusion is relatively resistant to neuroleptics and to stopping alcohol and can result in physical attacks on the partner or even homicide. Fortunately, onset is rare in old age. Sometimes, where there is also alcoholic dementia, an incomplete form of the syndrome occurs that may be more amenable to treatment.

The problem of defining the limits of "safe" drinking for elderly people has already been touched upon. Some evidence suggests that even for younger people "social drinking" may not be entirely safe as it can affect problem solving, abstraction, memory, and psychomotor function.[69,80] Any problems are likely to be magnified by the effects of age. A *severity-continuum* hypothesis suggests that cognitive deficit varies from absent or barely detectable in social drinkers through to Korsakoff psychosis and alcoholic dementia in very heavy drinkers.[81] The elderly population may be more at risk and the role of alcohol in cognitive impairment may be difficult to disentangle from that of normal aging,[69] not to mention that of coexistent Alzheimer's disease or vascular brain damage.

Management

Public Health Measures

There is good evidence that harm from alcohol consumption is linked to national drinking habits,[82] and this applies across all age groups. More than 20 years ago the Royal College of Psychiatrists' Report on Alcohol and Alcoholism[6] made firm recommendations concerning prevention. It proposed that national per capita consumption should not be allowed to rise and that agreement should be reached to bring alcohol consumption down over the following decade with concurrent monitoring of indices of harm (e.g., road traffic accidents involving alcohol and deaths from alcoholic cirrhosis). Other recommendations included coordinated efforts by different government departments to use public revenue policies to achieve these aims and a greatly enhanced commitment to education, persuasion, and relevant research. At a community and personal level, employers and individuals were asked to review the extent to which work and social activities press people to drink more than is good for them. Special efforts were advised for those trades and professions known to be at risk. Sadly, despite initiatives at the community level, vested interests have made it difficult to achieve anything at the political level.

In old age, bereavement, retirement, and loneliness may precipitate late-onset alcohol abuse.[63] To tackle these problems, improved leisure and activity opportunities with a healthier social attitude to bereavement (and counseling for those who need it) are needed. Many elderly people who abuse alcohol are dependent on other people for their supplies. Sometimes there may be several helpers supplying alcohol, each unaware of the others.[63,83] Public education is therefore needed to promote the message that excessive drinking in old age is not a harmless foible but a source of damage and disability. Doctors need educating too. Medical personnel[84] and psychiatric trainees[85] have been shown to take inadequate drinking histories given the known high prevalence of alcohol problems in medical and psychiatric inpatients.[86] Doctors were less likely to take adequate alcohol histories in women, although there is no evidence that they take less thorough histories in older people.[87] More recently, an Australian study has shown better alcohol histories with doctors taking an adequate history in 74% and nurses in 71%, increasing to 77 and 79% after two years of a New South Wales government nursing initiative on the nursing management of alcohol and other drugs.[88] If necessary, a history from other informants should be sought, as well as asking the patient specifically about alcohol consumption. A home visit can often reveal important clues in the form of half-empty glasses and empty bottles or self-neglect.

Suspicion should also be especially high in patients presenting with unexplained confusion, repeated falls, and atypical affective illness or where close relatives are known to be abusing alcohol.[63] Questionnaires that have not been specifically validated in the elderly population are not substitutes for a proper alcohol history.

Treatment

Acute Phase

Often, a great deal of preliminary work has to be done to detect alcohol abuse and bring the patient to a point where he or she acknowledges the problem. When alcohol abuse is established, and the patient is willing, treatment should begin with alcohol withdrawal. Often this will be on an inpatient basis since physical illness, especially pneumonia, peptic ulceration, and, rarely but importantly, subdural hematoma may complicate alcohol withdrawal. Because these problems may be present atypically in elderly people, it is particularly important to be aware of them. In view of the risk of the Wernicke–Korsakoff syndrome and other complications of poor nutrition and vitamin deficiency, early vitamin supplementation is essential, usually with high-potency parenteral B and C preparations. Oral preparations should subsequently be continued. In patients who have been drinking heavily immediately before coming into the hospital, withdrawal symptoms (and the risk of delirium tremens) should be minimized by the use of a decreasing regime of chlormethiazole or chlordiazepoxide, although some would advise against chlordiazepoxide in view of its long half-life.[68] Oral chlormethiazole should be given in reduced dosage in older people[36] and in those with cirrhosis.[89] Hypokalemia, dehydration, and other electrolyte imbalances should be corrected, if necessary, by intravenous (IV) infusion.[90] Hypoglycemia can accompany withdrawal and may be corrected by IV injection of glucose although IV thiamine should be given at the same time to prevent precipitation of Wernicke's encephalopathy. Sympathetic nursing in an appropriately lighted and controlled environment is essential during this phase. Functional psychiatric symptoms such as depression or psychotic phenomena need treatment in their own right, but care has to be taken when using drugs that may lower the epileptic threshold, already low in alcohol withdrawal. Indeed, some would advise routine use of antiepileptic drugs as part of the alcohol withdrawal regime. Chronic subdural hematoma should be suspected where there is an unexpected degree of confusion, especially if there is marked diurnal or even hour-to-hour fluctuation in the level of consciousness. Acute subdural hematoma presents with coma. In either case, an urgent CT scan and neurosurgical assessment are indicated. The pain of alcoholic neuropathy, which may not respond to conventional analgesics, may be amenable to treatment with carbamazepine. Recently, a pilot study has explored the possibility of alcohol withdrawal at home for frail elderly people.[91] This should be attempted only when adequate resources and medical supervision are available to recognize and manage any complications.

Continuing Care and Prognosis

When drinking is of late onset, in response to remediable social stress, the prognosis is relatively good, especially if the patient and relatives acknowledge the problem. Detailed restructuring of the social network can remove both the need and the opportunity for heavy drinking.[63] Often, there is also a need to educate the patient and caregivers about the alcohol contents of different drinks and about the effects of alcohol upon the elderly person. At this stage of treatment, the emphasis is on social and educational intervention rather than on medical treatment using drugs such as disulfiram, which may be dangerous in older people.[68] Where excessive drinking is more longstanding, prognosis is not so good. Where there is collusion by other alcoholic individuals (including family members) using the elderly person's money as a source of supply, prognosis may be especially poor unless the patient can be removed from that situation.[63]

In many countries, including the U.K., mental health legislation for compulsory treatment specifically excludes alcohol problems, although intervention is allowed if secondary mental illness supervenes. It may be that elder-abuse legislation (now common in the U.S.) will help in the situation where an elderly person is being encouraged to drink excessively as part of an exploitative situation. Where brain damage impairs judgment, deliberate restriction of alcohol supply through institutional care may be the only way to prevent further damage. As long ago as 1964, Droller[83] suggested that treated elderly alcoholic individuals should be discharged to a communal living situation such as residential care.

Conclusion

Medical and social services face a challenge from the increasing number of old and very old people who sometimes have multiple illnesses and dependency. Excessive alcohol consumption is an avoidable and treatable cause of illness and dependency. It is relatively rare in old age but is likely to become more common as a result of the aging of the population, social changes in drinking habits, cohort effects, and relative affluence, especially among "young" elderly people in many societies. Its small but significant contribution to the overall burden of dependency should be recognized. In individual terms, too, the recognition and appropriate treatment of alcohol abuse can produce dramatic benefit.

References

1. Atkinson, R., Aging and alcohol use disorders: diagnostic issues in the elderly, *Int. Psychogeriatr.*, 2, 55, 1990.
2. Adams, W.L., Barry, K.L., and Fleming, M.F., Screening for problem drinking in older primary care patients, *J. Am. Med. Assoc.*, 276, 1964, 1996.
3. Schuckit, M.A., Daeppen, J.B., Tipp, J.E., Hesselbrock, M., and Bucholz, K.K., The clinical course of alcohol-related problems in alcohol dependent and non-alcohol dependent drinking men and women, *J. Stud. Alcohol.*, 59, 581, 1998.
4. *Diagnostic and Statistical Manual of Mental Disorders: DSM-IV*, American Psychiatric Association, Washington, D.C., 1994.
5. *The ICD-10 Classification of Mental and Behavioural Disorders: Clinical Descriptions and Diagnostic Guidelines.* World Health Organisation, Geneva, 1992.
6. Royal College of Psychiatrists, *Alcohol and Alcoholism*, Tavistock Publications, London, 1979.
7. Mishara, B.L. and Kastenbaum, R., *Alcohol and Old Age*, Grune and Stratton, London, 1992.
8. Smart, R.G., Behavioural and social consequences related to the consumption of different beverage types, *J. Stud. Alcohol.*, 57, 77, 1996.
9. Levenson, M.R., Aldwin, C.M., and Spiro, A., Age, cohort and period effects on alcohol consumption and problem drinking: findings from the Normative Aging Study, *J. Stud. Alcohol.*, 59, 712, 1998.
10. Knupfer, G. and Room, R., Abstainers in a metropolitan community, *Q. J. Stud. Alcohol.*, 31, 108, 1970.
11. Cartwright, A.K., Shaw, S.J., and Spratley, T.A., The relationships between per capita consumption, drinking patterns and alcohol-related problems in a population sample. 1965–1974. 1. Increased consumption and changes in drinking patterns, *Br. J. Addict.*, 73, 237, 1978.
12. Busby, W.J., Campbell, A.J., Borrie, M.J., and Spears, G.F., Alcohol use in a community-based sample of subjects aged 70 years and older, *J. Am. Geriatr. Soc.*, 36, 301, 1988.
13. Dunne, F.J., Misuse of alcohol or drugs by elderly people, *Br. Med. J.*, 308, 608, 1994.
14. Adams, W.L. and Cox, N.S., Epidemiology of problem drinking among elderly people, *Int. J. Addict.*, 30, 1693, 1995.
15. Mirand, A.L. and Welte, J.W., Alcohol consumption among the elderly in a general population, Erie County, New York, *Am. J. Public Health*, 86, 978, 1996.
16. Fink, A., Hays, R.D., Moore, A.A., and Beck, J.C., Alcohol-related problems in older persons. Determinants, consequences and screening, *Arch. Intern. Med.*, 156, 1150, 1996.
17. McInnes, E. and Powell, J., Drug and alcohol referrals: are elderly substance abuse diagnoses and referrals being missed? *Br. Med. J.*, 308, 444, 1994.
18. Adams, W.L., Alcohol use in retirement communities, *J. Am. Geriatr. Soc.*, 44, 1082, 1996.
19. Barker, J.C. and Kramer, B.J., Alcohol consumption amongst older urban American Indians, *J. Stud. Alcohol.*, 57, 119, 1996.

20. Hirata, E.S., Almeida, O.P., Funari, R.R., and Klein, E.L., Alcoholism in a geriatric outpatient clinic of Sao Paulo, Brazil, *Int. Psychogeriatr.*, 9, 95, 1997.

21. Lakhani, N., Alcohol use amongst community-dwelling elderly people: a review of the literature, *J. Adv. Nurs.*, 25, 1227, 1997.

22. Edwards, G., Hawker, A., Hensman, C., Peto, J., and Williamson, V., Alcoholics known or unknown to agencies: epidemiological studies in a London suburb, *Br. J. Psychiatr.*, 123, 169, 1973.

23. Bridgewater, R., Leigh, S., James, O.F.W., and Potter, J.F., Alcohol consumption in elderly patients in an urban community, *Br. Med. J.*, 295, 884, 1987.

24. Iliffe, S., Haines, A., Booroff, A., Goldenberg, E., Morgan, P., and Gallivan, S., Alcohol consumption by elderly people: a general practice survey, *Age Ageing*, 20, 120, 1991.

25. Saunders, P.A., Copeland, J.R.M., Dewey, M.E., Davidson, I.A., McWilliam, C., Sharma, V., and Sullivan, C., Heavy drinking as a risk factor for depression and dementia in elderly men: findings from the Liverpool longitudinal community study, *Br. J. Psychiatr.*, 159, 213, 1991.

26. Prescott, C.A., Hewitt, J.K., Truett, K.R., Heath, A.C., Neale, M.C., and Eaves, L.J., Genetic and environmental influences on lifetime alcohol-related problems in a volunteer sample of older twins, *J. Stud. Alcohol.*, 55, 184, 1994.

27. Gorman, D.M., Is the disease model an appropriate term to describe the alcohol dependence syndrome? *Alcohol Alcohol.*, 24, 509, 1989.

28. Murray, R., Alcoholism, in *Essentials in Postgraduate Psychiatry*, Hill, P., Murray, R., and Thorley, A., Eds., Grune and Stratton, London, 1986, p. 324.

29. Rosin, A.J. and Glatt, M.M., Alcohol excess in the elderly, *Q. J. Stud. Alcohol.*, 32, 53, 1971.

30. Atkinson, R., Late onset problem drinking in older adults, *Int. J. Geriatr. Psychiatr.*, 9, 321, 1994.

31. Hauser, J. and Rybakowski, J., Three clusters of male alcoholics, *Drug Alcohol Dependency*, 48, 243, 1997.

32. Liberto, J.G., Oslin, D.W., and Ruskin, P.E., Alcoholism in older persons: a review of the literature, *Hosp. Community Psychiatr.*, 43, 975, 1992.

33. Vestal, R.E., McGuire, E.A., Tobin, J.D., Andres, R., Norris, A.H., and Mezey, R., Aging and ethanol metabolism in man, *Clin. Pharmacol. Ther.*, 3, 343, 1977.

34. Helderman, J.H., Vestal, R.E., Rowe, J.W., Tobin, J.D., Andres, R., and Robertson, G., The response of arginine vasopressin to intravenous alcohol and hypertonic saline in man: the impact of ageing, *J. Gerontol.*, 33, 39, 1978.

35. Walker, J. and Wynne, H., Review: the frequency and severity of adverse drug reactions in elderly people, *Age Ageing*, 23, 255, 1994.

36. Ramsay, L.E. and Tucker, G.T., Drugs and the elderly, *Br. Med. J.*, 282, 125, 1981.

37. Neve, R.J., Lemmens, P.H., and Drop, M.J., Drinking careers of older male alcoholics in treatment as compared to younger alcoholics and to older social drinkers, *J. Stud. Alcohol.*, 58, 303, 1997.

38. Mellstrom, D., Rundgren, A., and Svanborg, A., Previous alcohol consumption and its consequences for ageing, morbidity and mortality in men aged 70–75, *Age Ageing*, 10, 277, 1981.

39. Marx, J., Alcohol and trauma, *Emerg. Med. Clin. North Am.*, 8, 929, 1990.

40. Groover, J.R., Alcoholic liver disease, *Emerg. Med. Clin. North Am.*, 8, 887, 1990.

41. MacMath, T.L., Alcohol and gastro-intestinal bleeding, *Emerg. Med. Clin. North Am.*, 8, 859, 1990.

42. Sternbach, G.L., Infections in alcoholic patients, *Emerg. Med. Clin. North Am.*, 8, 793, 1990.
43. Peacock, W.F., Cardiac disease in the alcoholic patient, *Emerg. Med. Clin. North Am.*, 8, 775, 1990.
44. Ragland, G., Electrolyte abnormalities in the alcoholic patient, *Emerg. Med. Clin. North Am.*, 8, 761, 1990.
45. Singh, M. and Simsek, H., Ethanol and the pancreas: current status, *Gastroenterology*, 98, 1051, 1990.
46. Barburiak, J.J. and Rooney, C.B., Alcohol and its effects on nutrition in the elderly, in *Handbook of Nutrition in the Aged*, Watson, R.R., Ed., Boca Raton, FL, CRC Press, 1985.
47. Dunne, F.J., Alcohol and the immune system, *Br. Med. J.*, 298, 543, 1989.
48. Scheig, R., Immunologic abnormalities in alcoholic liver disease, *Am. J. Gastroenterol.*, 85, 371, 1990.
49. Stemmerman, G.N., Nomwa, A.M., Chyon, P.H., and Yoshizawa, C., Prospective study of alcohol intake and large bowel cancer, *Dig. Dis. Sci.*, 35, 1414, 1990.
50. La Vecchia, C., Negri, E., Parazzini, F., Boyle, P., Fasoli, M., Gentile, A., and Franceschi, S., Alcohol and breast cancer: update from an Italian case-control study, *Eur. J. Cancer Clin. Oncol.*, 25, 1711, 1989.
51. Hiatt, R.A., Alcohol consumption and breast cancer, *Med. Oncol. Tumor Pharmacother.*, 7, 143, 1990.
52. Garaglioni, C.F., Lilienfield, A.M., and Mendeloff, A.I., Incidence rates of liver cirrhosis and related diseases in Baltimore and selected areas of the United States, *J. Chronic Dis.*, 32, 543, 1979.
53. Aron, E., Dupin, M., and Joberd, P., Les cirrhoses du trosieme age, *Ann. Gastroenterol. Hepatol.*, 15, 558, 1979.
54. Potter, J.F. and James, O.W.F., Clinical features and prognosis of alcoholic liver disease in respect of advancing age, *Gerontology*, 33, 380, 1987.
55. Klatsky, A.L., Armstrong, M.A., and Friedman, G.D., Risk of cardiovascular mortality in alcohol drinkers, ex-drinkers and non-drinkers, *Am. J. Cardiol.*, 66, 1237, 1990.
56. Gronbaek, M., Deis, A., Sorensen, T.I., Becker, U., Borch-Johnsen, K., Muller, C., Schnohr, P., and Jensen, G., Influence of sex, age, body mass index, and smoking on alcohol intake and mortality, *Br. Med. J.*, 308, 302, 1994.
57. Rubino, F.A., Neurologic complications of alcoholism, *Psychiatr. Clin. North. Am.*, 15, 359, 1992.
58. Lishman, W.A., Alcohol and the brain, *Br. J. Psychiatr.*, 56, 635, 1990.
59. Marco, C.A. and Kelen, G.D., Acute intoxication, *Emerg. Med. Clin. North Am.*, 8, 731, 1990.
60. Perkin, G.D. and Hondler, C.E., Wernicke-Korsakoff syndrome, *Br. J. Hosp. Med.*, 30, 331, 1983.
61. Foy, A., Kay, J., and Taylor, A., The course of alcohol withdrawal in a general hospital, *QJM*, 90, 253, 1997.
62. Joyce, E.M., Aetiology of alcoholic brain damage: alcoholic neurotoxicity or thiamine malnutrition? *Br. Med. Bull.*, 50, 99, 1994.
63. Wattis, J.P., Alcohol problems in the elderly, *J. Am. Geriatr. Soc.*, 3, 131, 1981.
64. Ron, M., Acker, W., Shaw, G.K., and Lishman, W.A., Computerised tomography of the brain in chronic alcoholism: a survey and follow-up study, *Brain*, 105, 497, 1982.

65. Mann, K., Mundle, G., Langle, G., and Petersen, D., The reversibility of alcoholic brain damage is not due to rehydration: a CT study, *Addiction*, 88, 649, 1993.
66. Jacobson, R., The contribution of sex and drinking history to the CT brain scan changes in alcoholics, *Psychol. Med.*, 16, 547, 1986.
67. Mann, K., Batra, A., Gunthner, A., and Schroth, G., Do women develop alcoholic brain damage more readily than men? *Alcohol. Clin. Exp. Res.*, 16, 1052, 1992.
68. Dunne, F.J. and Schipperheijn, J.A., Alcohol and the elderly, *Br. Med. J.*, 298, 1660, 1989.
69. Grant, I., Adams, K.M., and Reed, R., Ageing, abstinence and medical risk factors in the prediction of neuropsychological deficit among long-term alcoholics, *Arch. Gen. Psychiatr.*, 41, 710, 1984.
70. Marmot, M.G., Elliott, P., Shipley, M.J., Dyer, A.R., Ueshima, H., Beevers, D.G., Stamler, R., Kesteloot, H., Rose, G., and Stamler, J., Alcohol and blood pressure: the INTERSALT study, *Br. Med. J.*, 308, 1263, 1994.
71. Rix, K.J., Alcoholism and the Elderly, master's thesis, Edinburgh University, 1980.
72. Gaitz, C.M. and Baer, P.E., Characteristics of elderly people with alcoholism, *Arch. Gen. Psychiatr.*, 24, 372, 1971.
73. Smith, D.M. and Atkinson, R.M., Alcoholism and dementia, *Int. J. Addict.*, 30, 1843, 1995.
74. Berlyne, N., Confabulation, *Br. J. Psychiatr.*, 120, 31, 1972.
75. Jacobson, R.R. and Lishman, W.A., Cortical-diencephalic lesions in Korsakoff's syndrome: a clinical and CT scan study, *Psychol. Med.*, 20, 63, 1990.
76. Victor, M., Adams, R.D., and Collins, G.H., *The Wernicke-Korsakoff Syndrome and Related Neurological Disorders Due to Alcoholism and Malnutrition*, 2nd ed., F.A. Davis, Philadelphia, 1989.
77. Cutting, J., The relationship between Korsakoff's syndrome and alcoholic dementia, *Br. J. Psychiatr.*, 132, 240, 1978.
78. Victor, M., Adams, R.D., and Mancall, E.L., A restricted form of cerebellar cortical degeneration occurring in alcoholic patients, *Arch. Neurol.*, 1, 579, 1959.
79. Harper, C. and Krill, J., Brain atrophy in chronic alcoholic patients: a quantitative pathological study, *J. Neurol. Neurosurg. Psychiatr.*, 48, 211, 1985.
80. Robertson, I., Does moderate drinking cause mental impairment? *Br. Med. J.*, 289, 711, 1984.
81. Parker, E.S. and Parker, D.A., Towards an epidemiology of cognitive deficits among alcohol consumers, in *Cerebral Deficits in Alcoholism*, Wilkinson, D.A., Ed., Addiction Research Foundation, Toronto, 1983.
82. Smith, R., The politics of alcohol, *Br. Med. J.*, 284, 1392, 1982.
83. Droller, H., Some aspects of alcoholism in the elderly, *Lancet*, 2, 137, 1964.
84. Barrison, I.G., Viola, L., and Murray-Lyon, I.M., Do housemen take an adequate drinking history? *Br. Med. J.*, 281, 1040, 1980.
85. Farrell, M.P. and David, A.S., Do psychiatric registrars take a proper drinking history? *Br. Med. J.*, 296, 395, 1988.
86. Jarman, C.M. and Kellett, J.M., Alcoholism in the general hospital, *Br. Med. J.*, 2, 469, 1979.
87. Awad, I. and Wattis, J.P., Alcohol histories in hospital: does the age and sex of the patient make a difference? *Br. J. Addict.*, 85, 149, 1990.
88. Burns, L. and Adams, R., Alcohol-history taking by nurses and doctors — how accurate are they really? *J. Adv. Nurs.*, 25, 509, 1997.

89. Pentikaunen, P.J., Neuvonen, P.J., Taspila, S., and Syvalahti, E., Effects of cirrhosis of the liver on the pharmacokinetics of chlormethiazole, *Br. Med. J.*, 2, 861, 1978.
90. Rix, K.J., Alcohol withdrawal states, *Hosp. Update*, 403, 1978.
91. Evans, D.J., Street, S.D., and Lynch, D.J., Alcohol withdrawal at home. Pilot project for frail elderly people, *Can. Fam. Physician*, 42, 937, 1996.

2

Cognitive Changes in Aging Alcoholics

Marlene Oscar-Berman and Patrick McNamara

CONTENTS

Introduction

Many researchers have noted a similarity in the brain changes observed with normal chronological aging and brain changes occurring after many years of alcoholism (reviewed by Oscar-Berman and colleagues[1,2]). For example, Wilkinson and Carlen[3] described a study in which brain scans of alcoholic individuals were compared to those of patients who had a variety of neurological conditions unrelated to alcoholism. The ages of all of the patients ranged from the 20s through the 60s. The researchers found that the brains of the alcoholic patients, as well as chronologically older nonalcoholic patients, appeared to be shrunken inside their skulls. Decades earlier, Courville[4] described this same feature of cerebral atrophy in the autopsied brain specimens of alcoholic individuals, and he likened it to the brain volume decrease that occurs with normal chronological aging. That is, alcoholic and normal aging individuals showed widespread cortical shrinkage, most prominently in the frontal part of the brain. Considered together, these findings provided early evidence that gave rise to the *premature aging hypothesis*, i.e., the idea that alcoholism somehow accelerates normal chronological aging.[5]

Because of the similarities in the brains of alcoholic and aging individuals, investigators began a search for parallels in functional decline. Consequent to this new research, reports appeared that noted similarities between alcoholic individuals and chronologically older normal controls in loss of cognitive abilities.[1,6] Both groups had difficulty with tasks that tap executive cognitive functions, as well as "nonverbal" visuospatial abilities as assessed by performance subtests of the Wechsler Adult Intelligence Scale[7] (WAIS). These observations led, independently, to models that implicate the same areas of brain involvement with alcoholism and with normal chronological aging. One such model suggests that alcoholism and aging are associated with decline in abilities mediated by prefrontal brain systems, and another suggests that the right half of the brain is more vulnerable to the effects of alcoholism — and to the effects of aging — than the left half of the brain.[2,8]

The present chapter examines evidence regarding each of the three hypotheses noted above, i.e., the premature aging hypothesis, the *frontal systems hypothesis*, and the *right hemisphere hypothesis*. Based upon the evidence, the following explanation for the differential vulnerability of frontal and right-sided brain systems in alcoholism and aging is proposed: With normal chronological aging and with alcoholism, brain structures embedded in the cytoarchitectonically and evolutionarily defined neuroanatomic regions known as the *archicortical trend* are most vulnerable. If alcoholism proceeds to a more extensive illness, such as alcoholic Korsakoff syndrome, then systems in other neuroanatomic regions known as the *paleocortical trend* become involved as well. Similarly for aging: The initial structures affected are those of the archicortical trend throughout the right hemisphere. If dementia becomes part of the picture, then structures of the paleocortical trend in both hemispheres also are affected. It is suggested that the right hemisphere is most affected initially in both alcoholism and aging because the systems of the archicortical trend (e.g., dorsolateral prefrontal, mesial and inferior temporal, superior parietal cortical areas, etc.) are more pronounced on the right than on the left. Furthermore, the ratio of white to gray matter on the right is greater in the archicortical system.[9] Since alcoholism and other degenerative processes are known to influence neuronal fibers (white matter) as well as cortex, initially right hemispheric brain regions are likely to be affected. The following discussion of evolutionary cytoarchitectonics provides a brief background to a review of the alcoholism and aging literature in which the premature aging hypothesis, the frontal systems hypothesis, and the right hemisphere hypothesis were considered.

Evolutionary Cytoarchitectonics and the Archicortical and Paleocortical Trends

Sanides[10,11] hypothesized that the cerebral cortex is ultimately derived from two primordial generative sites or moieties: an archicortex (hippocampus) and a paleocortex (olfactory cortex). From each of these primitive allocortices, Sanides and later investigators[12,13] traced a trend of cortical differentiation characterized by the progressive development of cortical laminae and passing from periallocortical areas to proisocortical areas and culminating in true six-layered isocortex. The archicortical moiety is the forerunner of isocortex on the medial surface of the hemisphere, whereas the paleocortical moiety gives rise to the isocortex on the ventral and lateral surfaces. Mesial temporal sites, for example, stem largely from the archicortical trend while the entire superior temporal gyrus and portions of the inferior temporal lobes emanate largely from the paleocortical trend. In the frontal lobes, the paleocortical trend originates in the temporal pole and adjacent orbital frontal region and gives rise to the isocortex on the ventral and ventrolateral frontal surfaces. The archicortical trend arises from proisocortex on the medial surface of the hemispheres and differentiates into dorsal and dorsolateral areas of the frontal lobes. A similar set of findings is obtained for each of the other regions of the hemispheres. The paleocortical trend gives rise to the face, neck, and head areas of the post-central somatic sensory areas (SI and portions of SSII), as well as portions of the inferior parietal lobule. Conversely, the archicortical trend gives rise to limb and trunk regions of the somatosensory strip, as well as rostral portions of SSII and the superior parietal lobule. In the visual areas, the paleocortical trend gives rise to the ventral visual system extending into the inferior temporal lobe with connections to the parahippocampal gyrus, while the archicortical trend proceeds anteriorly into the superior parietal sites. Pandya and colleagues[13] suggested that, in general, the systems of the paleocortical trend function to answer the question, "What is it?" while the archicortical division, whether it appears in anterior or posterior regions of the cortex, answers the question, "Where is it?"

Alcoholism and Premature Aging

As noted earlier, similarities in neuropathological and neuropsychological consequences of alcoholism and aging led to the premature aging hypothesis. The premature aging hypothesis has been put forth in two versions.[6] According to the first version, the *accelerated aging* (or *cumulative effects*) model, alcoholism is accompanied by the precocious onset of neuroanatomical and behavioral changes typically associated with advancing age. Cognitively, or neuropsychologically, alcoholic individuals become old before their time. The second version places the timing of the changes somewhat differently. According to this view, which has been labeled the "increased vulnerability" model, the aging brain is more vulnerable to the harmful effects of alcoholism than is the brain of a younger person. Therefore, the cognitive decline associated with normal chronological aging (beginning at around age 50) receives added momentum when combined with alcoholism. This version proposes that older alcoholic individuals are impaired compared with age-matched nonalcoholic individuals; however, this would not be the case for younger alcoholic individuals.

Taken together, most of the evidence from neuropathological and neuro-imaging investigations supports the view of a link between alcoholism and premature aging. Furthermore, studies favoring the increased vulnerability model are more common than those supporting the accelerated aging model. Elderly alcoholic individuals have an increased risk of toxicity and side effects (including accidents) resulting from alcohol intake. In part, this is because older people have a decreased ability to metabolize alcohol, and they may have concomitant medical problems.[14] As predicted by the increased vulnerability model, certain brain structures show greater reduction in size in older alcoholic than in younger alcoholic individuals. These are the cerebral cortex,[15] the corpus callosum,[16] the hippocampus[17] (but see Reference 18), and the cerebellum.[19-21] Recent findings from magnetic resonance imaging (MRI) studies also have shown increased brain tissue loss in alcoholic compared with nonalcoholic individuals, even after their ages had been taken into account.

Results of neurobehavioral investigations tend to support the view that aging increases one's vulnerability to alcohol-related decline, but controversy prevails because the association between alcoholism and aging has been less reliable with behavioral measures than with imaging techniques.[1,22] More importantly, when neuroradiological and behavioral changes are examined together in the same study, concomitant brain damage with performance impairments is not always found. For example, Sullivan and colleagues[20] reported clear evidence of brain abnormalities but no differences on explicit memory tests in alcoholic individuals relative to nonalcoholic controls ages 21 to 70. Explicit memory refers to the ability to remember facts and events consciously; it is assessed by recognition and recall tests, and is impaired in alcoholic Korsakoff and other amnesic patients.[23-25] The hippocampus and adjacent cortical areas have been strongly implicated in explicit memory by a host of neuropsychological, brain imaging, and nonhuman animal studies.[26] Sullivan et al.[20] evaluated whether or not there were correlations between MRI measures of hippocampal volume and behavioral measures of verbal and nonverbal memory. Anterior portions of the hippocampus were found to be smaller in alcoholic individuals than in controls, and this difference was even greater in older than in younger alcoholic individuals. While the MRI findings supported the increased vulnerability model, the behavioral significance of the neuroanatomical reduction (i.e., increased hippocampal vulnerability in aging and alcoholism) was unclear because the explicit memory scores did not correlate with hippocampal volumes. Indeed, the alcoholic individuals were not impaired on the memory tests. Further, although Sullivan et al.[20] observed visuospatial impairments on an IQ subtest that has a memory component (Digit Symbol), they observed no significant correlations with hippocampal volume.

In contrast to the Sullivan et al.[20] findings were those from another study that found no evidence of cortical atrophy but did show aging-related cognitive deficits.[27] In that study, older alcoholic individuals and controls were given MRI scans and numerous age-normed neuropsychological tests to compare brain measures and cognitive abilities. The alcoholic individuals displayed clear impairments on memory and visuospatial tasks, but there were no group differences in global cerebral atrophy (although two did have significant atrophy). One reason for cognitive dysfunction in the absence of changes in gross brain morphology is that synaptic neuronal alterations that affect processing exist but are undetectable at a macroscopic anatomical scale.[28] However, Di Sclafani et al.[27] did find a stronger association between age and ventricular dilation in the alcoholic individuals than in the controls (as did Pfefferbaum and colleagues[29]).

In a neurobehavioral study, Ellis[30] found that alcoholic individuals ages 48 to 74 were impaired compared with nonalcoholic peers and younger alcoholic individuals (ages 25 to 47) on performance IQ subtests of the WAIS. Although that finding was supportive of the increased vulnerability hypothesis, another observation in the same study was not supportive. The older alcoholic individuals did not show deficits out of proportion to their age on dichotic listening tasks of right hemisphere functioning (a string of piano notes). In another study assessing the cognitive domain of selective attention,[31] male and female alcoholic individuals and nonalcoholic controls between ages 29 and 76, were given a cued-detection task in which the pre-cue provided information about the most probable visual-field (VF) location of a subsequent target letter. The nonalcoholic controls showed a VF asymmetry, reflected as a specific disruption when the cue was presented in the right VF and the target was presented in the left VF. Unlike the younger control subjects, the alcoholic individuals in both age groups (and the older nonalcoholic controls) showed no evidence of a right hemisphere (left VF) advantage on the task; they were influenced by the validity of the cue regardless of the visual field in which it was presented. In sum, within the cognitive domain of selective attentional processing, the results from this experiment provided support for the accelerated aging model of premature aging (and also for the right hemisphere model discussed later).

Involvement of Cerebral Cortex and Frontal Brain Systems

It was noted earlier that certain brain structures — notably the cerebral cortex, hippocampus, and cerebellum — show greater reduction in size in older alcoholic than in younger alcoholic individuals.[15,17,21,27,29] In this section, changes in the cerebral cortex are emphasized. With chronic alcoholism as well as with aging, cortical changes have been reported throughout the brain, but there is consistent evidence that some cortical regions, especially in the frontal lobes, are especially vulnerable.[20,32-38]

In a series of studies conducted early in our research efforts, we assessed frontal integrity in a simple and direct way: We used classical delayed reaction tasks such as delayed response (DR) and delayed alternation (DA).[39,40] Delayed reaction tasks have special sensitivity to frontal system damage, especially deficits in working memory and response inhibition. Abnormal perseverative responding (the inability to inhibit unintended responses) is thought to underlie the deficits of patients with frontal disorders on many tasks, including delayed reaction tasks. Furthermore, successful performance on DR and DA tasks is known to rely upon different underlying neuroanatomical and neuropsychological mechanisms. Thus, the prefrontal cortex is host to at least two subsystems: dorsolateral and orbitofrontal. Although the dorsolateral system contains intimate connections with other neocortical sites, its connections with limbic sites are less striking than those of the orbitofrontal system. The dorsolateral system, although important for successful performance on both DR and DA, is especially important for DR performance, in which visuospatial, mnemonic, and attentional functions are considered critical. By contrast, functions involved in response inhibition have been linked to the orbitofrontal system. The orbitofrontal system is intimately connected with basal forebrain and limbic structures; its connections with other neocortical regions are not as extensive as those of the dorsolateral system. The orbitofrontal system, like the dorsolateral system, supports successful performance on both DA and DR, but it is especially important for DA performance. Results of our early studies indicated that both of these frontal systems are affected by alcoholic Korsakoff disease. However, the tasks were not sufficiently sensitive to disclose deficits in alcoholic individuals without Korsakoff syndrome, nor in aging individuals.

Consequently, in another set of experiments with alcoholic and aging subjects, we measured frontal-system functions using sensitive computer-automated auditory and visual DR tasks.[41] By measuring reaction times as well as accuracy, and by manipulating stimulus durations (20 to 500 ms) as well as delays between stimuli and choices (0 to 30 s), we assessed separate component functions simultaneously: strategy learning, stimulus processing time, and short-term memory, respectively. We tested alcoholic men (including a group with Korsakoff syndrome) and nonalcoholic controls. The controls and the non-Korsakoff alcoholic men were equated for age within two age brackets: young, which we defined as up to age 49, and older, which we defined as 50 and over. Those four subgroups formed the basis for one set of statistics looking at the separate contributions of aging and alcoholism. The age range of the group with Korsakoff syndrome was 52 to 68 years. Therefore, we matched them with non-Korsakoff alcoholic men and controls of similar ages.

All of the groups of subjects were able to learn the simple task of pressing the left lever for one color or sound, and pressing the other lever for a different color or sound. Also, they all benefited equally from having the spatial cue available; in other words, the spatial tasks were easier than the nonspatial tasks. However, there were important group differences. Although the non-Korsakoff alcoholic men and the same-age controls did not differ from each other, the patients with Korsakoff syndrome were impaired. Whether the DR task was presented in the visual or the auditory modality, the patients with Korsakoff syndrome were less proficient than their age-matched peers. Impairments by the patients with Korsakoff syndrome became exaggerated as demands were placed on short-term memory (long delay intervals, over 15 s) and on visual processing time (brief exposures, up to about 80 ms). In other words, not only did the patients with Korsakoff syndrome display their classic short-term memory deficit, they also did not process incoming information as fast as the other subjects. These results parallel findings reported in earlier studies of visual processing and memory deficits of patients with Korsakoff syndrome performing other delay tasks (e.g., delayed matching-to-sample short term[42] and delayed nonmatching-to-sample[43]).

What about the detoxified alcoholic men who do not have Korsakoff syndrome, i.e., the four age-matched groups of non-Korsakoff alcoholic men and normals? Here we were looking for possible age effects from the groups in which we had a wider age range to work with than the subjects with Korsakoff syndrome. We also looked for alcohol effects with larger groups of alcoholic and normal individuals matched for age. We found quite a bit of overlap among the four subgroups. Overall, however, the older subjects (whether or not they had a history of alcoholism) showed deficits in processing and in short-term memory (although their deficits were not nearly so dramatic as those of the patients with Korsakoff syndrome). Older subjects generally performed more poorly than younger subjects under the most difficult conditions, but these differences were absent in the easier conditions.

There were two instances in which the older alcoholic men showed the biggest deficits. For example, in the auditory modality only, the older alcoholic men were significantly less accurate than the young alcoholic men at the shortest delay, and in one visual DR condition, the older normal men were faster to respond than older alcoholic men. The additive effects of alcoholism and aging were small, however, and the results that were statistically significant were based on combined data for many of the experimental parameters. Nonetheless, these instances provided some support for the age sensitivity version of the premature aging hypothesis that places emphasis on the appearance of alcohol-related deficits in the older age range.

These results were confirmed by many subsequent findings that semantic, procedural, or implicit memories are relatively spared in alcoholic amnesia, but that declarative, episodic, or explicit memories are especially vulnerable.[25,44] As we reported for the experiment using older subjects with the automated DR procedures, on delayed-matching and delayed-nonmatching tasks, older individuals were impaired compared with younger alcoholic individuals and nonalcoholic controls, and the age-related differences were exaggerated in the alcoholic individuals.

Functional and structural neuroimaging techniques also have revealed frontal abnormalities in alcoholic individuals. Investigators have reported finding reduced metabolic activity in the frontal lobes, as well as in cingulate, parietal, parieto-occipital, and mesial temporal regions[45-48] and significantly smaller gray and/or white matter volume.[49,50] Selective neuronal loss in the frontal lobes has also been observed at a microscopic level.[35] Additionally, Pfefferbaum and colleagues[29] conducted regional MRI analyses of cortical integrity and found evidence that cortical volume loss in alcoholism and aging is selective. The frontal lobes were especially vulnerable to chronic alcoholism at any age, but the effects were exacerbated in elderly people; temporal-parietal loss occurred mainly in aged alcoholic individuals. Another recent study[50] showed fewer regional abnormalities, but the investigators did note a loss of white matter in the posterior superior temporal region that also had been noted in the study by Pfefferbaum et al.[29]

Some studies of frontal lobe function with older alcoholic individuals have confirmed reports of a correlation between impaired neuropsychological performance on tests of frontal functioning (e.g., executive control skills) and decreased frontal lobe perfusion or metabolism.[32,45] In contrast, in another study, researchers obtained cerebral blood flow measures and computerized tomography (CT) scans in a sample of 40 patients with chronic alcoholism, and related the neuroradiological findings to the results of neuropsychological testing.[51] The researchers found evidence of significant brain hypoperfusion in the alcoholic individuals. In 26 of the 40, the reduced blood flow was mainly in the frontal lobes, but only about 25% of them (11 of the 40) had CT evidence of frontal atrophy. Furthermore, the alcoholic individuals exhibited significant impairments on tests of frontal lobe functioning and visuospatial skills.

Working memory functions in the dorsolateral frontal cortex are thought to affect posterior processing, thereby influencing posterior activity. Therefore, vulnerable frontal neural systems that support working memory in alcoholic individuals may exert an impaired influence on right posterior regions of the brain as well. We suggest that posterior — as well as frontal — neural systems may be impaired in alcoholic individuals, especially those over the age of 50. Regardless, it is clear that short-term, working memory for visuospatial information is impaired. Given the neuroanatomical links between short- and long-term memory functions,[52] there are strong ramifications regarding long-term memory impairments in alcoholism and aging. Impairment of long-term memory for visuospatial information may thus result to some extent from impaired visuospatial working memory, as well as impaired visuospatial processing.

Involvement of the Right Hemisphere

The mental tasks that alcoholic and aging individuals have difficulty with also are similar to the kinds of tasks that patients with damage to the right hemisphere encounter with difficulty. The observations led, independently, to what is known as the *right hemisphere hypothesis* in both the alcoholism literature and the aging literature.[8] The hypothesis developed separately within each subdiscipline, and the relevance to the premature aging hypothesis (which had derived from similarities in alcoholic and aging subjects) was not immediately apparent. The right hemisphere hypothesis states simply that the right half of the brain might be more vulnerable to the effects of alcoholism (or to the effects of aging) than the left half of the brain. In other words, the disproportionate decline in nonverbal, visuospatial functions (noted earlier) was attributed to a greater sensitivity of the right hemisphere to the biological onslaught of alcoholism or aging.

In our laboratory, we tested the right hemisphere hypothesis directly, by employing tasks sensitive to functional asymmetries of the two cerebral hemispheres.[1,6] As a class, these tasks are referred to as dichotomous stimulation tasks. They rely upon the simultaneous inputs from two separate sensory channels on the left and the right sides of the body — the two ears, or the two visual half-fields, or the two hands, for example. Mainly because of the organization of the brain, with language lateralized to the left hemisphere, and nonlanguage lateralized more or less to the right (along with numerous crossed connections of sensory fields with contralateral brain areas), under dichotomous input conditions (with competing inputs from the right and left sides of the body), the right input channel is better than the left when "verbal" (linguistic) stimulus materials are used, and the left side is superior to the right with "nonverbal" (visuospatial, musical) stimulus materials. In a series of many studies, we gave the dichotomous stimulation tests in three different sensory input modalities, vision, touch, and audition.[53] Although we obtained support for the premature aging hypothesis from several studies, the evidence was not overwhelming. Thus, in a few instances, we did observe greater deficits in alcoholic men over the age of 50 than in their age-matched nonalcoholic controls. We concluded that the brains of people over age 50 may be somewhat abnormally susceptible to the effects of alcohol, as the age sensitivity version of the hypothesis posits, but it is not a large effect. Results of dichotomous stimulation studies did not support the hypothesis that alcoholism differentially affects right hemisphere functions.

Nor did they support the hypothesis that normal chronological aging differentially affects right hemisphere functions. Similarly, no differential hemispheric effects were observed for the combined effects of alcoholism and aging.

In sum, the findings have not been sufficiently consistent to resolve the premature aging issue; there is only equivocal support for the hypothesis that either alcoholism or aging differentially affects the functioning of the two cerebral hemispheres.[1,6,53-55] The early emphasis on defective nonverbal performance may have been an artifact of at least two features of the nonverbal tasks employed: (1) perceptual processing demands, and (2) the need to formulate new, effective strategies for getting information into short-term memory. Most simple verbal tasks (including verbal IQ tests), because they can be easily processed, tended to be approached with simple strategies. Nonverbal tasks, by contrast, typically employ materials that are far less familiar than words, and require more time to be processed and the use of new elaborate strategies for problem solution. However, when enough processing time was given, and when strategies were simplified in one way or another, alcoholic and aging subjects were able to perform on nonverbal tasks as well as they could perform on verbal tasks. Their overall performance levels often were lower than younger subjects — just as they were in some of the DR tasks, and probably for the same reasons — but not because of greater right- than left-hemisphere decline. When patients with Korsakoff syndrome were tested on dichotomous stimulation tasks, they showed the same asymmetries as the other groups, but their overall levels of performance were even lower than the others' — just as they were in the DR tasks.

Musical, Facial, and Emotional Cognition

The topic of right hemisphere integrity is important not just from the standpoint of contributions to visuospatial cognitive functions, but also because of the role of the right hemisphere in other neuropsychological processes. In addition to spatial cognition, other functions under control of the right hemisphere might be expected to be disrupted according to an archicortical right hemisphere hypothesis of alcoholism. Among the functions with strong right hemisphere involvement are musical, facial, and affective cognition. Note that whereas spatial cognition may be related to configural (or global) analysis of faces,[56] spatial ability (such as that measured by mental rotation) and emotion are not related.[57] Ellis[30] found that dichotically presented tonal patterns were processed similarly by alcoholic individuals and controls but not by patients with right hemisphere lesions. This finding is to be expected by our hypothesis since the tones would have been handled by superior temporal (i.e., paleocortical) networks — not by archicortical networks. By contrast, in another study of dichotic perception of melodies and words, alcoholic men did show evidence of right hemisphere dysfunction: they had a significantly smaller left-ear superiority for melodies, and a significantly larger right-ear superiority for words than controls.[58]

Pictures of faces comprise another stimulus material that is dominated by right hemisphere processing. Moreover, convergent findings in cognitive neuroscience indicate that right hemisphere specialization for face stimuli takes place in low-level visual perceptual and higher-order semantic and other cognitive systems.[59-61] Thus, nearly any task with face stimuli should probe right hemisphere dominant brain functions, making faces an especially crucial material for testing the right hemisphere hypothesis of alcoholism and aging. However, since cognitive neuroscientific evidence implicates the paleocortically derived right posterior ventral region in face perception,[61] and by our hypothesis these paleocortical visual areas are not impaired in alcoholism, face perception studies in alcoholic individuals should lead largely to null results. There is, in fact, a dearth of evidence for alcoholic brain damage specific to this region, and null results are typical in this area of study.[62,63] While alcoholic patients with Korsakoff syndrome, who have long-term explicit memory impairments (for recent evidence see Reference 64), are deficient at perceiving and remembering the emotional information conveyed by faces, non-Korsakoff alcoholic individuals are not.[63] Elderly people, however, regardless of alcohol history, perceived and remembered fewer emotional expressions in the faces than younger people.[63] In contrast, another study found that alcoholic individuals correctly recognize fewer inverted faces than nonalcoholic controls.[65] Inverted faces, however, are thought to be processed by posterior brain areas on either the right or left involved in object perception rather than those areas critical for face perception; only upright faces benefit from processing in brain areas specialized for face perception.[66]

Emotional abnormalities such as those known to accompany alcoholism[63,67] result from lesions in multiple brain systems.[68-70] Modular models of emotion combine concepts from lateral dominance with ideas about cortical-subcortical interactions.[68] Many brain centers act to take in emotional cues, evaluate them, and execute appropriate reactions. Nonetheless, the role of the right hemisphere in emotional functions generally is more relevant than that of the left. Emotional changes known to accompany long-term chronic alcoholism resemble the emotional changes characteristic of patients with right hemisphere damage.[63,67] Events that normally would hold emotional significance may elicit no emotional response in these patients, who, in addition, might generate little spontaneous emotionally oriented behavior. Interpersonally, certain alcoholic individuals, like patients with right hemisphere damage, leave an impression of dullness, apathy, or emotional flatness that may be mistaken for depression. Talland,[71] in describing a possible mechanism for the severe memory loss accompanying alcoholic Korsakoff syndrome, commented that the patient's failure to sustain emotional involvement in ongoing events was an important factor.

The right hemisphere (especially in the right frontal lobe) is more relevant for processing negative emotions than positive emotions.[68,69] Therefore, tasks that measure emotional functions (especially tasks that include stimuli with a negative valence) can be used to tap right hemisphere abilities. If alcoholic individuals have deficient right hemisphere function, they should have more difficulty perceiving emotional materials than nonemotional materials. Moreover, among the emotional materials, alcoholic individuals should have more difficulty perceiving negative than positive emotional stimuli. Likewise, if alcoholism interacts with aging, then deficits should be most pronounced in older alcoholic individuals (compared with their nonalcoholic peers). On the other hand, if emotion depends more on paleocortically derived orbitofrontal regions than on archicortically derived dorsolateral regions, then, by an archicortical hypothesis, emotional processing in alcoholism may not be significantly impaired.

In a study of emotional functions in alcoholic individuals in our laboratory, a visual backward-masking and perceptual laterality paradigm was used to assess emotional processing abilities in detoxified alcoholic individuals compared with nonalcoholic controls aged 30 to 69 years.[72] Emotional and nonemotional words were presented to the left or right VFs, followed by a visual masking stimulus. The research participants were asked to judge the emotional valence of each word (positive, negative, or neutral) and to respond verbally or manually (button presses). The dependent measure was the critical interstimulus interval needed to escape the backward-masking effect. The alcoholic individuals showed a significant right VF (left hemisphere) advantage in both response modes, whereas the controls did not. Furthermore, older alcoholic individuals showed a selective impairment in processing negative words. Thus, when emotional materials were used, the findings supported the claim that alcoholic individuals suffer some right hemispheric impairment relative to healthy controls and that this right hemispheric impairment impedes some aspects of emotional processing. More global tests of emotional comprehension and emotional expression may disclose little or no differences between alcoholic individuals and controls.[1,54,55]

In another study from our laboratory,[73] we used variations of the Stroop color-word interference task to assess emotional abilities in alcoholic individuals and nonalcoholic controls across a wide age span (29 to 83 years). We presented positive and negative emotional words, and neutral words, in a color-naming paradigm; i.e., the participants were asked to report only the colors of the words, which were written in different colored inks. We hypothesized that if there are changes in emotional perception as a function of alcoholism and/or aging, then alcoholic individuals (especially those over age 50) would show abnormal interference effects for emotional as compared with neutral words, and negative words might be less disruptive than positive words. Results showed expected emotional interference effects for all subjects, and differences in emotional valence processing were found among older subgroups: Older alcoholic individuals were more susceptible than older nonalcoholic controls to the interference effects, and positive emotional words produced a greater interference effect than negative and neutral words. Thus, the findings provided some support for the right hemisphere hypothesis (as well as for the premature aging hypothesis).

In sum, while the pattern of neurocognitive decline associated with alcoholism and with aging consistently implicates right hemispheric decline in visuospatial tasks, the impairments are not generalizable to all skill sets that are known to depend on right hemisphere structural integrity. Athough fewer studies of emotional abnormalities have been reported in the literature on alcoholism and aging than studies of dichotomous hemispheric asymmetries, it appears that the right hemisphere hypothesis explains emotional abnormalities somewhat better than it explains deficits in visuospatial cognitive functions. It may be that age and alcoholism-related neurological changes affect sites in both hemispheres but that right hemisphere systems are more extensively affected than left hemisphere systems. In addition, it is probably the case that certain systems within the right hemisphere are more affected than others.

Summary and Conclusions

The cerebral cortex shows greater reduction in size in older alcoholic than in younger alcoholic individuals.[15,17,21,27,29] With chronic alcoholism as well as with aging, cortical changes have been reported throughout the brain, but there is consistent evidence that some regions, especially cortex in the frontal lobes and cortex throughout the entire right hemisphere, may be especially vulnerable. This chapter reviewed changes in the cerebral cortex in relation to possible synergistic effects of alcoholism and aging.

With respect to frontal lobe systems, research has demonstrated that alcoholic patients with Korsakoff syndrome are considerably more vulnerable to damage in these regions than normal aging and alcoholic subjects without Korsakoff syndrome. For the latter groups, results of neuroimaging studies have consistently demonstrated abnormalities, but neurobehavioral findings have been mixed.

The right and left halves of the brain process sensory input and motor information differently. Whereas the left hemisphere has a dominant role in linguistic behavior and the right hemisphere plays a dominant role in spatial cognition and emotional behaviors, the two hemispheres are complementary in their processing modes depending upon context and task demands. The left hemisphere plays a special role in processing piecemeal information analytically and sequentially, and the right hemisphere plays a special role in integrating information holistically. A common observation in work with alcoholic and with normal aging individuals is that both groups show lower scores on performance IQ subtests (containing many visuospatial tasks) than on verbal IQ subtests. From these observations, several hypotheses have emerged: (1) alcoholism may affect right hemispheric functions more than left hemispheric functions; (2) aging may affect right hemispheric functions more than left hemispheric functions; and (3) alcoholism may accelerate normal chronological aging. Research on cognitive capabilities and differences between the two cerebral hemispheres in alcoholic and in nonalcoholic aging individuals has provided only limited support for the premature aging hypothesis, and even less consistent support for the right hemisphere hypothesis.

Based upon a review of neuropsychological and neuroimaging studies, we have suggested a unifying neuroanatomic hypothesis of alcoholism and of aging that explains many aspects of the neurocognitive changes. With normal chronological aging, as with alcoholism, brain structures embedded in the archicortical trend are initially most vulnerable; the first structures affected are those of the archicortical trend throughout the right hemisphere. If alcoholism is accompanied by Korsakoff syndrome, or if dementia occurs with aging, then systems in the paleocortical trend in both hemispheres are affected as well. In general, findings from evolutionary and architectonic analyses of cortical structure provide a reasonable explanation for the facts concerning neurocognitive consequences of alcoholism and aging, and certain findings are compatible with the right hemisphere hypothesis as well. Nonetheless, several caveats are in order.

First, each of the two architectonically defined evolutionary trends gives rise to three subdivisions within each sensorimotor cortical region. These are called the root, core, and belt regions. Generally, core regions correspond to primary sensory or primary motor regions, root regions correspond to supplementary cortices, and belt regions correspond to association areas. It may be that alcoholism predominantly affects one of these three regions within the archicortical trend. Data as yet do not allow this issue to be decided. Second, our hypothesis does not rule out damage to paleocortical systems. We suggest only that archicortical trends are predominantly affected primarily because they are first affected. Finally, we have not discussed subcortical connectivity patterns of the two above-described cytoarchitectonic trends, but subcortical systems clearly are affected by alcoholism.[21] The evidence suggests, however, that there is a greater involvement of subcortical systems linked to the archicortical (e.g., hippocampus and paralimbic sites) than to the paleocortical trend systems.

Since distinct functions and multiple brain areas can underlie different cognitive tasks, broadly defined neurobehavioral alterations can occur from injury to only a subset of structures. Cognitive neuroscientific research has made notable progress in recent years with the advent of new functional brain imaging techniques and improvements to traditional neurobehavioral approaches to understanding brain systems involved in human behaviors. These findings with populations of neurologically intact and impaired nonalcoholic individuals, coupled with the neuroanatomical, neuropsychological, and cognitive neuroscientific studies of alcoholic and elderly individuals, have provided additional means for precisely testing the premature aging hypothesis and the frontal and right hemisphere hypotheses. To date, the increased vulnerability model of the premature aging hypothesis has received more support from imaging research than from neurobehavioral research. However, conclusive support still has not been forthcoming for either hypothesis.

Nonetheless, with the new techniques available, we anticipate a successful future in understanding the ways the cerebral hemispheres act to integrate and complement their functions, as well as a similar leap in progress at pinpointing precisely the neurobehavioral consequences of long-term chronic alcoholism, normal chronological aging, and the synergism of alcoholism and aging. Identification of distinct neurofunctional systems that are differentially affected in alcoholism and cognitive aging is crucial for development of rational therapeutic strategies that can ameliorate or prevent the destruction of these systems. The evidence reviewed in this chapter suggests that the archicortical system is especially important in this regard.

Acknowledgment

The writing of this chapter was supported by funds from the U.S. Department of Health and Human Services, National Institute on Alcohol Abuse and Alcoholism (R37-AA07112 and K05-00219), and by funds from the Medical Research Service of the U.S. Department of Veterans Affairs.

References

1. Oscar-Berman, M. and Schendan, H.E., Asymmetries of brain function in alcoholism: relationship to aging, in *Neurobehavior of Language and Cognition: Studies of Normal Aging and Brain Damage*, Obler, L. and Connor, L.T., Eds., Kluwer Academic Publishers, New York, 2000, 215–240.
2. Oscar-Berman, M., Neuropsychological vulnerabilities in chronic alcoholism, in Review of NIAAA's *Neuroscience and Behavioral Research Portfolio*, Noronha, A., Eckardt, M., and Warrant, K., Eds., Monograph No. 34, NIAAA, NIH, USDHHS, 2000, Rockville, MD, 1999.
3. Wilkinson, D.A. and Carlen, P.L., Morphological abnormalities in the brains of alcoholics: relationship to age, psychological test scores and patient type, in *Alcoholism and Aging: Advances in Research*, Wood, W.G. and Elias, M.F., Eds., CRC Press, Boca Raton, FL, 1982, 61–77.
4. Courville, C.B., *Effects of Alcohol on the Nervous System of Man*, 2nd ed., San Lucas Press, Los Angeles, 1966.
5. Parsons, O.A., Sinha, R., and Williams, H.L., Relationships between neuropsychological test performance and event-related potentials in alcoholic and nonalcoholic samples, *Alcohol. Clin. Exp. Res.*, 14, 746–755, 1990.

6. Ellis, R.J. and Oscar-Berman, M., Alcoholism, aging, and functional cerebral asymmetries, *Psychol. Bull.*, 106, 128–147, 1989.
7. Wechsler, D., *Wechsler Adult Intelligence Scale–Revised: Manual*, The Psychological Corporation, New York, 1981.
8. Parsons, O., Neuropsychological consequences of alcohol abuse: many questions — some answers, in *Neuropsychology of Alcoholism*, Parsons, O., Butters, N., and Nathan, P., Eds., Guilford Press, New York, 1987, 153–175.
9. Gur, R.C., Packer, I.K., Hungerbuhler, J.P. et al., Differences in the distribution of gray and white manner in human cerebral hemispheres, *Science*, 207, 1226–1228, 1980.
10. Sanides, F., Functional architecture of motor and sensory cortices in primates in light of a new concept of neocortex evolution, in *The Primate Brain: Advances in Primatology*, Noback, C.R. and Montagna, W., Eds., Meredith Corp., New York, 1970, 137–208.
11. Sanides, F., Representation in the cerebral cortex and its areal lamination pattern, in *The Structure and Function of Nervous Tissue*, Bourne, G.H., Ed., Academic Press, New York, 1972, 329–453.
12. Barbas, H., Anatomic basis of cognitive-emotional interactions in the primate prefrontal cortex; *Neurosci. Behav. Rev.*, 19, 499–510, 1995.
13. Pandya, D.N., Seltzer, B., and Barbas, H., Input-output organization of the primate cerebral cortex, in *Comparative Primate Biology*, Vol. 4, Steklis, H.D. and Erwin, J., Eds., Alan R. Liss, New York, 1988, 39–80.
14. National Institute on Alcohol Abuse and Alcoholism, Ninth Special Report to the U.S. Congress on Alcohol and Health, Bethesda, MD, NIAAA, 1997.
15. Nicolás, J.M., Estruch, R., Salamero, M. et al., Brain impairment in well-nourished chronic alcoholics is related to ethanol intake, *Ann. Neurol.*, 41, 590–598, 1997.
16. Pfefferbaum, A., Lim, K.O., Desmond, J.E., and Sullivan, E.V., Thinning of the corpus callosum in older alcoholic men: a magnetic resonance imaging study, *Alcohol. Clin. Exp. Res.*, 20, 752–757, 1996.
17. Sullivan, E.V., Deshmukh, A., Desmond, J.E. et al., Volumetric MRI analysis of cerebellar hemispheres and vermis in chronic alcoholics: relationship to ataxia (abstr.), *J. Int. Neuropsychol. Soc.*, 2, 34, 1996.
18. Harding, A.J., Wong, A., Svoboda, M., Kril, J.J., and Halliday, G.M., Chronic alcohol consumption does not cause hippocampal neuron loss in humans, *Hippocampus*, 7, 78–87, 1997.
19. Harris, G.J., Oscar-Berman, M., Gansler, D.A., Streeter, C., Lewis, R.F., Ahmed, I., and Achong, D., Hypoperfusion of the cerebellum and aging effects on cerebral cortex blood flow in abstinent alcoholics: a SPECT study, *Alcohol. Clin. Exp. Res.*, 23, 1219–1227, 1999.
20. Sullivan, E.V., Marsh, L., Mathalon, D.H., Lim, K.O., and Pfefferbaum, A., Anterior hippocampal volume deficits in nonamnesic, aging chronic alcoholics, *Alcohol. Clin. Exp. Res.*, 19, 110–122, 1995.
21. Sullivan, E.V., Neuropsychological vulnerabilies in chronic alcoholism, in *Review of NIAAA's Neuroscience and Behavioral Research Portfolio*, Noronha, A., Eckardt, M., and Warrant, K., Eds., Research Monograph No. 35, Publication No. 99, National Institute on Alcohol Abuse and Alcoholism, Rockville, MD, 1999.

22. Evert, D.L. and Oscar-Berman, M., Alcohol-related cognitive impairments: an overview of how alcoholism may affect the workings of the brain, *Alcohol Health Res. World*, 19, 89–96, 1995.
23. Kopelman, M.D., The Korsakoff syndrome, *Br. J. Psychiatr.*, 166, 154–173, 1995.
24. Mayes, A.R., Memory and amnesia, *Behav. Brain Res.*, 66, 29–36, 1995.
25. Oscar-Berman, M. and Evert, D.L. Alcoholic Korsakoff's syndrome, in *Handbook of Neuropsychology and Aging*, Nussbaum, P.D., Ed., Plenum, New York, 1997, 201–215.
26. Eichenbau, H., Declarative memory: insights from cognitive neurobiology, *Annu. Rev. Psychol.*, 48, 547–572, 1997.
27. Di Sclafani, V., Ezekiel, F., Meyerhoff, D.J. et al., Brain atrophy and cognitive function in older abstinent alcoholic men, *Alcohol. Clin. Exp. Res.*, 19, 1121–1126, 1995.
28. Harper, C., The neuropathology of alcohol-specific brain damage, or does alcohol damage the brain? *J. Neuropathol. Exp. Neurol.*, 57, 101–110, 1998.
29. Pfefferbaum, A., Sullivan, E.V., Mathalon, D.H., and Lim, K.O., Frontal lobe volume loss observed with magnetic resonance imaging in older chronic alcoholics, *Alcohol. Clin. Exp. Res.*, 21, 521–529, 1997.
30. Ellis, R.J., Dichotic asymmetries in aging and alcoholic subjects, *Alcohol. Clin. Exp. Res.*, 14, 863–971, 1990.
31. Evert, D. and Oscar-Berman, M., Selective attentional processing and the right hemisphere: effects of alcoholism and aging, submitted.
32. Adams, K.M., Gilman, S., Johnson-Greene, D. et al., The significance of family history status in relation to neuropsychological test performance and cerebral glucose metabolism studied with positron emission tomography in older alcoholic patients, *Alcohol. Clin. Exp. Res.*, 22, 105–110, 1998.
33. Davila, M.D., Shear, P.K., Lane, B., Sullivan, E.V., and Pfefferbaum, A., Mammillary body and cerebellar shrinkage in chronic alcoholics: an MRI and neuropsychological study, *Neuropsychology*, 8, 433–444, 1994.
34. Estruch, R., Nicolas, J.M., Salamero, M. et al., Atrophy of the corpus callosum in chronic alcoholism, *J. Neurol. Sci.*, 146, 145–151, 1997.
35. Kril, J.J., Halliday, G.M., Svoboda, M.D., and Cartwright, H., The cerebral cortex is damaged in chronic alcoholics, *Neuroscience*, 79, 983–998, 1997.
36. Pfefferbaum, A. and Rosenbloom, M.J., *In vivo* imaging of morphological brain alterations associated with alcoholism, in *Alcohol-Induced Brain Damage*, Hunt, W.A. and Nixon, S.J., Eds., NIAAA Research Monograph No. 22, Publication No. 93-3549. Rockville, MD, USDHHS, National Institutes of Health, 1993, 71–87.
37. Shear, P.K., Sullivan, E.V., Lane, B., and Pfefferbaum, A., Mammillary body and cerebellar shrinkage in chronic alcoholics with and without amnesia, *Alcohol. Clin. Exp. Res.*, 20, 1489–1495, 1996.
38. Wang, G.J., Volkow, N.D., Roque, C.T. et al., Functional importance of ventricular enlargement and cortical atrophy in healthy subjects and alcoholics as assessed with PET, MR imaging, and neuropsychologic testing, *Radiology*, 186, 59–65, 1993.
39. Freedman, M. and Oscar-Berman, M.N., Bilateral frontal lobe disease and selective delayed response deficits in humans, *Behav. Neurosci.*, 100, 337–342, 1986.

40. Oscar-Berman, M., McNamara, P., and Freedman, M., Delayed-response tasks: parallels between experimental ablation studies and findings in patients with frontal lesions, in *Frontal Lobe Function and Dysfunction*, Levin, H.S., Eisenberg, H.M., and Benton, A.L., Eds., Oxford University Press, New York, 1991, 230–255.

41. Oscar-Berman, M., Hunter, N., and Bonner, R.T., Visual and auditory spatial and nonspatial delayed-response performance by Korsakoff and non-Korsakoff alcoholic and aging individuals, *Behav. Neurosci.*, 106, 613–622, 1992.

42. Oscar-Berman, M. and Bonner, R.T., Matching- and delayed matching-to-sample performance as measures of visual processing, selective attention, and memory in aging and alcoholic individuals, *Neuropsychologia*, 23, 639–651, 1985.

43. Oscar-Berman, M. and Bonner, R.T., Nonmatching- (oddity) and delayed non-matching-to-sample performance in aging, alcoholic, and alcoholic Korsakoff individuals, *Psychobiology*, 17, 424–430, 1989.

44. Oscar-Berman, M. and Bardenhagen, F., Nonhuman primate models of memory dysfunction in neurodegenerative disease: contributions from comparative neuropsychology, in *Memory in Neurodegenerative Disease*, Tröster, A., Ed., Cambridge University Press, New York, 1998, 3–20.

45. Adams, K.M., Gilman, S., Koeppe, R.A. et al., Neuropsychological deficits are correlated with frontal hypometabolism in positron emission tomography studies of older alcoholic patients, *Alcohol. Clin. Exp. Res.*, 17, 205–210, 1993.

46. Gansler, D.A., Harris, G.J., Oscar-Berman, M. et al., Hypoperfusion of inferior frontal brain regions in abstinent alcoholics: a pilot SPECT study, *J. Stud. Alcohol*, 61, 32–37, 2000.

47. Gilman, S., Koeppe, R.A., Adams, K.M. et al., Positron emission tomographic studies of cerebral benzodiazepine-receptor binding in chronic alcoholics, *Ann. Neurol.*, 40, 163–171, 1996.

48. Volkow, N.D., Wang, G.J., Begleiter, H. et al., Regional brain metabolic response to lorazepam in subjects at risk for alcoholism, *Alcohol. Clin. Exp. Res.*, 19, 510–516, 1995.

49. Jernigan, T.L., Butters, N., DiTraglia, G. et al., Reduced cerebral grey matter observed in alcoholics using magnetic resonance imaging, *Alcohol. Clin. Exp. Res.*, 15, 418–427, 1991.

50. Sullivan, E.V., Mathalon, D.H., Lim, K.O., Marsh, L., and Pfefferbaum, A., Patterns of regional cortical dysmorphology distinguishing schizophrenia and chronic alcoholism, *Biol. Psychiatr.*, 43, 118–131, 1998.

51. Nixolás, J.M., Catafau, A.M., Estruch, R. et al., Regional cerebral blood flow-SPECT in chronic alcoholism: relation to neuropsychological testing, *J. Nucl. Med.*, 34, 1452–1459, 1993.

52. Gabrieli, J.D.E., Desmond, J.E., Demb, J.B. et al., Functional magnetic resonance imaging of semantic memory processes in the frontal lobes, *Psychol. Sci.*, 7, 278–283, 1996.

53. Oscar-Berman, M., Alcoholism and asymmetries of brain function, *Alcohol Health Res. World*, 16, 273–279, 1992.

54. Bates, M.E. and Convit, A., Neuropsychology and neuroimaging of alcohol and illicit drug abuse, in *The Assessment of Neuropsychological Functions in Psychiatric Disorders*, Calev, A., Ed., American Psychiatric Press, Washington, D.C., 373–345, 1999.

55. Rourke, S.B. and Løberg, T., The neurobehavioral correlates of alcoholism, in *Neuropsychological Assessment of Neuropsychiatric Disorders*, 2nd ed., Grant, I. and Nixon, S.J., Eds., Oxford University Press, New York, 1996, 423–485.
56. Tanaka, J.W. and Farah, M.J., Parts and wholes in face recognition, *Q. J. Exp. Psychol. Hum. Exp. Psychol.*, 46A, 225–245, 1993.
57. Crucian, G.P. and Berenbaum, S.A., Sex differences in right hemisphere tasks, *Brain Cognition*, 36, 377–389, 1998.
58. Drake, A.I., Hannay, H.J., and Gam, J., Effects of chronic alcoholism on hemispheric functioning: an examination of gender differences for cognitive and dichotic listening tasks, *J. Clin. Exp. Neuropsychol.*, 12, 781–797, 1990.
59. Buckner, R.L., Beyond HERA: contributions of specific prefrontal brain areas to long-term memory retrieval, *Psychol. Bull. Rev.*, 3, 149–158, 1996.
60. Damasio, H., Grabowski, T.J., Tranel, D., Hichwa, R.D., and Damasio, A.R., A neural basis for lexical retrieval, *Nature*, 380, 499–505, 1996.
61. Puce, A., Allison, T., Asgari, M., Core, J.C., and McCarthy, G., Differential sensitivity of human visual cortex to faces, letterstrings, and textures: a functional magnetic resonance imaging study, *J. Neurosci.*, 16, 5205–5215, 1996.
62. Cermak, L.S., Verfaellie, M., Letourneau, L. et al., Verbal and nonverbal right hemisphere processing by chronic alcoholics, *Alcohol. Clin. Exp. Res.*, 13, 611–661, 1989.
63. Oscar-Berman, M., Hancock, M., Mildworf, B., and Hunter, N., Emotional perception and memory in alcoholism and aging, *Alcohol. Clin. Exp. Res.*, 14, 383–393, 1990.
64. Oscar-Berman, M. and Pulaski, J.L., Associative learning and recognition memory in alcoholic Korsakoff patients, *Neuropsychology*, 11, 282–289, 1997.
65. Nixon, S.J. and Bowlby, D., Evidence of alcohol-related efficiency deficits in an episodic learning task, *Alcohol. Clin. Exp. Res.*, 20, 21–24, 1996.
66. Farah, M.J., Wilson, K.D., Drain, H.M., and Tanaka, J.R., The inverted face inversion effect in prosopagnosia: evidence for mandatory, face-specific perceptual mechanisms, *Vision Res.*, 35, 2089–2093, 1995.
67. Oscar-Berman, M., The contribution of emotional and motivational abnormalities to cognitive deficits in alcoholism and aging, in *Neuropsychology of Memory*, 2nd ed., Squire, L. and Butters, N., Eds., Guilford Press, New York, 1992, 81–94.
68. Borod, J.C., Cerebral mechanisms underlying facial, prosodic, and lexical emotional expression: a review of neuropsychological studies and methodological issues, *Neuropsychology*, 7, 445–463, 1993.
69. Gainotti, G., Caltagirone, C., and Zocolotti, P., Left/right and cortical/subcortical dichotomies in the neuropsychological study of human emotions, *Cognition Emotion*, 7, 71–93, 1993.
70. Heller, W., Nitschke, J.B., and Miller, G.A., Lateralization in emotion and emotional disorders, *Curr. Directions Psychol. Sci.*, 7, 26–32, 1998.
71. Talland, G.A., *Deranged Memory: A Psychonomic Study of the Amnesic Syndrome*, Academic Press, San Diego, CA, 1965.
72. Hutner, N. and Oscar-Berman, M., Visual laterality patterns for the perception of emotional words in alcoholic and aging individuals, *J. Stud. Alcohol.*, 57, 144–154, 1996.
73. Covall, S., Attentional and emotional processing in aging and alcoholism, Ph.D. dissertation, Behavioral Neuroscience Ph.D. Program, Boston University School of Medicine, Boston, MA, 1996.

3

Alcohol and the Heart in Humans and Animal Models

Michael J. Dunn, Vinood B. Patel, Victor R. Preedy,
Peter J. Richardson, and Simon Worrall

CONTENTS

Introduction

This chapter describes the pathogenesis of alcoholic heart muscle disease as a problem of cumulative alcohol intake, rather than due to immediate consumption or the type of alcohol beverage. Therefore, alcoholic heart muscle disease should be considered in terms of a problem occurring from middle to old age and the chapter is written from this perspective. However, the pathogenic mechanisms are unknown and the availability of clinical material for detailed biochemical analysis is limited. There is also considerable patient variability. This has led to the utilization of animal studies to provide sufficient material for elucidating the biochemical features and mechanisms of heart muscle damage in alcoholic cardiomyopathy. This chapter also describes three features of alcoholic cardiomyopathy, namely, the formation of acetaldehyde adducts, changes in cardiac enzyme activities, and protein analysis by two-dimensional polyacrylamide gel electrophoresis (2-DE). Comparative reference is made with observations derived from patient-based studies and experimental animals.

Cumulative Ethanol Intake as a Causative Factor of Alcoholic Cardiomyopathy

Although there is evidence that light to moderate drinking (1 to 4 drinks a day) is cardioprotective, there are substantial data supporting the contention that drinking alcohol in amounts greater than those recommended by the Royal Colleges in the U.K. is deleterious. Approximately one third of chronic alcohol misusers develop the disease entity *alcoholic cardiomyopathy*. Myocardial derangements for this disease include atrial fibrillation, early left ventricular diastolic dysfunction, and altered tissue biochemistry.[1] Ejection fractions are also impaired.[2,3] Many of the overt clinical features of alcoholic cardiomyopathy and dilated cardiomyopathy are indistinguishable, apart from the history of alcohol misuse in the former. However, a distinction between the two entities can be made at the histomorphological level.[1] At one time, a rule of thumb identified susceptible subjects with alcoholic cardiomyopathy as having consumed alcohol for approximately 10 years or more, at an average rate exceeding 80 g ethanol/day or a cumulative intake of 250 kg.[5] However, although this is a gross generalization, studies in Spain have investigated the importance of cumulative ethanol intake in more detail.[2,3] In these studies, ejection fractions were significantly correlated with cumulative ethanol intakes (reviewed in Reference 3). Inspection of the regression line shows that in men ejection fractions of 55% are obtained when cumulative intakes are 22 kg/ethanol kg body weight, equivalent to a lifetime intake of 1540 kg ethanol for the average 70-kg man.[2] This is much higher than the 250 kg originally proposed.[5] However, inspection of the Spanish data shows that 7 of the 52 male subjects studied had ejection fractions of 55% or less when cumulative alcohol consumption was between 7 and 20 kg/kg (490 and 1400 kg lifetime intake). It is important, nevertheless, to distinguish between functional and histomorphological parameters in the diagnosis of alcoholic cardiomyopathy. It is quite possible that histochemical or biochemical features of alcoholic cardiomyopathy may occur when cumulative alcohol intake is less than 500 kg, thus reaffirming the original definition of Richardson relating to the presence of alcoholic myopathy when cumulative ethanol intake exceeds 250 kg.[6] After reinterpreting the original definition for the occurrence of alcoholic cardiomyopathy, one should certainly inspect for alcoholic cardiomyopathy when cumulative alcohol intake is greater than 250 kg.

Given the cumulative feature of alcoholic cardiomyopathy, it is thus not surprising that this disease is infrequently seen in subjects younger than 40 years of age.[7] Thus generally, subjects studied are older than 40 years. For example, one study on alcoholic cardiomyopathy, had subjects with a mean age of 57 years who had consumed alcohol at a daily rate of 60 g ethanol for an average of 25 years (cumulative intake of 550 kg[8]).

Limitations in Patient Sample Availability and the Use of Animal Models

Although the pathological features of alcoholic cardiomyopathy are relatively well characterized, the precise causative mechanisms are unknown although some processes have been proposed. These include the involvement of altered membrane (i.e., sarcolemmal) integrity, damage by reactive oxygen species, changes in protein breakdown, and alterations in protein synthesis (reviewed in References 9 through 13).

As mentioned in the introduction to this chapter, it is very difficult to determine the precise biochemical effects of alcohol on the heart in patients because of limitation in sample availability and variation in patient population. Consequently, direct studies are usually carried out on hearts taken at autopsy (for example, see References 14 through 17) and only a few investigations have utilized samples taken by endomyocardial biopsy.[6,18-21] Furthermore, in patient-based studies, nutritional intake varies among alcohol misusers. This makes the data difficult to interpret as malnutrition also causes defined cardiac changes. These difficulties have led to the development of the Lieber–DeCarli regimen, although its original usage was in the field of alcoholic liver disease.[22,23] In this model, both control and treated animal groups receive identical amounts of dietary components, including micronutrients (such as trace elements and minerals) and macronutrients (such as lipids, carbohydrates, and protein), albeit with differences in calories provided as either ethanol (treated) or glucose or dextrin-maltose (controls). Thus, the possible involvement of dietary deficiencies in the etiology of alcoholic cardiomyopathy is negated.

Many of the histochemical features in hearts of patients with alcoholic cardiomyopathy are reproduced in the animal model, which include features of myofibrillary lysis, separation, and disintegration.[24-26] Scattered foci of lesions (e.g., fibrosis) and loss of parallel array are also observed in alcohol-fed laboratory animals: the severity of these lesions is enhanced with elevations in alcohol intake.[24-27] With the Lieber–DeCarli feeding regimen (which includes the element of pair-feeding to circumvent criticism that data are obtained as a result of malnutrition), left ventricle weights of alcohol-fed rats are increased at 4 to 11 months alcohol feeding, thus mimicking the cardio-megaly seen clinically.[28] However, although no overt changes in heart weights are seen at six to eight weeks, there are significant reductions in the contractile protein contents,[28,29] which are also seen clinically. The authors feel that the model employing a 6-week alcohol feeding regimen therefore represents a suitable means of examining the pathogenesis of cardiomyopathy.

There are only a few studies that have investigated the influences of age in the development of cardiac problems due to alcohol toxicity. Thus, in controlled studies comparing the effects of alcohol on the heart in young and old animals, a greater degree of cardiomegaly was reported in the older animals,[30] although indices of oxidative stress (cardiac lipofuscin deposits) were apparently lower.[31] Another study showed that in aged rats, much higher concentrations of ethanol are required *in vitro* to suppress peak tension development in isolated papillary muscle in older rats compared with younger animals.[32] These somewhat paradoxical data may arise because old rats are exposed to alcohol for the first time, whereas in the clinical situation cardiomyopathy develops over very long periods. To address this discrepancy, one needs to emphasize that alcoholic cardiomyopathy is a cumulative problem, and models should employ young animals and treat them for a long period to mimic the clinical situation.

The following synopsis focuses on three areas that have helped elucidate some of the pathogenic mechanisms involved in the etiology of alcoholic heart muscle damage. Clinical studies and laboratory animal studies are compared and contrasted.

Formation of Protein Adducts

By virtue of the extreme chemical reactivity of acetaldehyde, it is able to bind irreversibly with proteins to form acetaldehyde–protein adducts. Although most of this work has been carried out in the liver (for example, see References 33 and 34), only one investigation has been carried out in subjects with alcoholic cardiomyopathy.[35] This study did not look for endogenous adducts within cardiac tissue but measured immunoreactivity with cardiac proteins modified by acetaldehyde *in vitro*. In the aforementioned study, 21 patients with histologically proven cardiomyopathy were examined and the data showed that 7 of these had IgA and IgG antibodies that reacted against reduced acetaldehyde–protein adducts.[35] However, the patient range was large, from 23 to 63 years (mean of 45 years) and no analysis was carried out on the relationship between the cumulative alcohol intake and the presence of these antibodies. Other studies have shown that IgA reactivity with acetaldehyde-modified proteins is elevated in alcoholics[36] and heavy drinkers[37] when compared with social drinkers. Furthermore, the study by Harcombe and colleagues[35] did not examine antibodies reacting with unreduced-acetaldehyde–protein adducts, nor those pertaining to other adducts, such as hydroxyethyl or malondialdehyde–related protein adducts which are also found in the liver of alcohol misusers.[38-40]

In animal studies, adducts were examined in hearts of rats fed the Lieber–DeCarli alcohol-feeding regimen. ELISA analysis showed that there were significantly increased amounts of unreduced acetaldehyde–protein ($P < 0.01$), reduced acetaldehyde–protein ($P < 0.01$), and malondialdehyde acetaldehyde–protein ($P = 0.01$) adducts (Figure 3.1). There was no evidence for increased malondialdehyde and α-hydroxyethyl–protein adducts ($P > 0.05$ in both instances Worrall et al., manuscript in preparation). These animal studies represent the first evidence for the ethanol-induced formation of acetaldehyde-related adduct formation in heart tissue. All three acetaldehyde adducts, i.e., reduced, unreduced, and malondialdehyde acetaldehyde adducts were present. The increase in malondialdehyde acetaldehyde–protein adducts suggest that alcohol caused lipid peroxidation, concomitantly with the generation of acetaldehyde. There is some evidence to support the phenomenon of cardiac-derived acetaldehyde production as a number of studies have identified cardiac alcohol dehydrogenase (ADH) activities.[41-45]

Long-standing adduct formation may have rendered cardiac proteins inoperative via covalent linkages, conformational changes, or induced autoimmune responses.[46,47] It is worth noting that acetaldehyde-derived adducts are cardiotoxic with the ability to induce endothelial TNF-alpha release and upregulate ICAM-1.[48] This may further exacerbate cardiac derangements in alcohol toxicity.

Enzymatic Alterations

Increases in the activities of a number of cardiac enzymes, including lactate dehydrogenase, alpha-ketoglutarate dehydrogenase, creatine kinase, and malic dehydrogenase activities are observed in cardiac biopsies of heavy drinkers (Table 3.1, data for alpha-hydroxybutyric dehydrogenase and lactate dehydrogenase not presented for brevity[6]). Increased enzyme activities correlate with reduced ejection fraction and cumulative alcohol intake.[6] However, this phenomenon seems to be enzyme specific as aspartate aminotransferase activities are not altered. The aforementioned increased enzyme activities may represent either a feature of cardiac impairment or an adaptive process.

We examined whether a similar phenomenon occurred in rats subjected to alcohol feeding for 6 weeks (Table 3.2). In normotensive Wistar Kyoto (WKY) rats, total creatine kinase and malate dehydrogenase activities remained unchanged in response to chronic alcohol administration, whereas aspartate aminotransferase activities increased (Table 3.2). However, when ethanol feeding was carried out in spontaneously hypertensive rats (SHR), there were significant increases in creatine kinase and malic dehydrogenase activities, although aspartate aminotransferase activity was not significantly affected (Table 3.2). These results, in SHR, are similar to the qualitative data

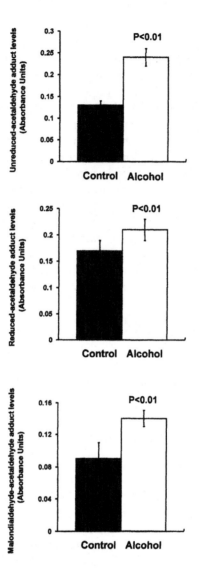

FIGURE 3.1
Reduced, unreduced, and malondialdehyde acetaldehyde–protein adducts in hearts of control and alcohol-fed rats. At the end of 6 weeks, hearts of rats fed either alcohol or isocaloric glucose were analyzed for protein adducts by ELISA. Data are expressed as absorbency units (405 nm for 10 µg tissue). All data are mean ± SEM (n = 6). NS, P > 0.05 not significant. Solid bars = control; open bars = ethanol. (Courtesy of Worrall et al.)

originally described by Richardson and colleagues.[6] However, the data contradict suggestions that reduced creatine kinase activity occurs in alcohol-feeding studies in rats.[49] Nevertheless, it seems that the concomitant pathology in alcoholism may influence the response of the cardiac enzymes. Certainly, the relationship between increasing alcohol intake and hypertension is well established.[50,51] In the study of Richardson et al.,[6] one third of patients

TABLE 3.1

Cardiac Enzyme Activities in Subjects Consuming Alcohol

| | Ethanol Consumption | | |
	Abstinent or Light	Heavy	P
Creatine kinase	1.67 + 0.13	2.72 + 0.22	<0.001
Malate dehydrogenase	2.09 + 0.19	2.98 + 0.19	<0.01
Aspartate aminotransferase	0.51 + 0.63	0.66 + 0.61	NS

Data as mean ± SEM, U/mg protein; NS = not significant. Light drinkers were defined as those who had a lifetime intake of less than 250 kg when daily intake exceeded 40 g per day (*n* = 13 for abstinent and light drinkers). Heavy drinkers exceeded 40 g per day and had a cumulative intake of 250 kg or more (*n* = 11).
Source: Adapted from Richardson et al. (1986).

(13/38) were hypertensive and significant correlations were obtained between blood pressure and cardiac creatine kinase activities ($P < 0.01$) and malate dehydrogenase ($P < 0.05$). However, exclusion of patients with hypertension also produced significant differences between cardiac enzyme activities in patients with light or heavy alcohol intake.[6]

Determination of myocardial enzymes can provide information on the current state of metabolic pathways, such as the citric acid cycle. Aspartate aminotransferase is an important enzyme involved in the malate/aspartate shuttle which transports reducing equivalents (i.e., NADH) and electrons from NADH into the mitochondria, which can then be utilized in the citric acid cycle or used for oxidative phosphorylation. However, there is some limitation in interpreting the data pertaining to these enzymes, as they frequently occur as isoenzymes. Thus, aspartate aminotransferase and malate dehydrogenase exist as two isoenzymes (found in the cytoplasm and mitochondria), whereas there are several isoenzymes of creatine kinase. However, there is a clear need to investigate the relationship between the pathogenesis of alcoholic cardiomyopathy and cardiac enzyme activities.

Proteomics

It is likely that significant alterations in the relative abundance of myocardial proteins occur in response to chronic alcohol consumption. Moreover, these changes may well determine the progression and outcome of the disease process. As described above, most previous biochemical studies of cardiac dysfunction in response to alcohol have been carried out on specific cellular systems. The alternative strategy is to investigate global alterations in cardiac protein expression, and this is now possible using the proteomic approach.

TABLE 3.2

The Effect of Chronic Alcohol Feeding on LV Cardiac
Enzyme Activities

		P
Creatine Kinase activity (U/mg DNA)		
WKY		
Control	26.7 ± 1.4	
Alcohol	28.0 ± 1.3	NS
SHR		
Control	20.5 ± 1.7	*
Alcohol	28.6 ± 1.7	<0.05
Malate Dehydrogenase Activity (U/mg DNA)		
WKY		
Control	36.1 ± 2.6	
Alcohol	39.0 ± 3.0	NS
SHR		
Control	33.8 ± 3.6	
Alcohol	42.8 ± 6.2	<0.05
Aspartate Aminotransferase (U/mg DNA)		
WKY		
Control	4.29 ± 0.54	
Alcohol	5.04 ± 0.33	<0.05
SHR		
Control	4.59 ± 0.52	
Alcohol	5.20 ± 0.30	NS

Male normotensive (WKY) and hypertensive (SHR) rats were studied at 16
weeks and fed alcohol as 35% of total calories (i.e., the Lieber–DeCarli regimen) for 6 weeks. Controls were pair-fed isocaloric glucose. All data are mean
± SEM of six observations. Differences between alcohol rats and correspond-
ing control pair-fed rats were assessed by Student's paired t-test, and P values
are indicated in the right-hand column. Differences between other means
were assessed by Student's t-test using the pooled estimate of variance. NS
= not significant.
* $P < 0.025$ for control SHR versus control WKY.

The term *proteome*, defined as the "PROTEin complement of the
genOME",[52] was initially applied to the characterization of whole organisms.
However, proteomics is now used in a narrower context to define patterns of
protein expression in particular cells and tissues. The first requirement for
proteome analysis is the separation of complex mixtures of proteins obtained
from whole tissues such as the heart. Currently, the best method is 2-DE,
which uses a combination of first-dimension separation by isoelectric focusing (IEF) under denaturing conditions with a second-dimension separation
by sodium dodecyl sulfate polyacrylamide gel electrophoresis (SDS-PAGE).

This orthogonal combination of a charge separation (isoelectric point, pI) with a size separation (molecular weight, MW) results in the sample proteins being distributed across the two-dimensional gel profile (Figure 3.2). Following 2-DE, the profiles of the separated proteins are visualized using a sensitive staining procedure (e.g., silver, fluorescence) and then digitized using an appropriate device (e.g., laser densitometer, CCD camera, fluorimager). Specialized, dedicated computer software is then used to derive qualitative and quantitative information from individual 2-D gels, to match the protein separation profiles from large numbers of 2-D gels and to construct comprehensive databases of quantitative protein expression. These databases can then be used to highlight changes in protein expression associated with a particular biological process. This process provides information on the abundance, pI, and MW of the separated proteins, but gives no direct clues as to their identities or functions. Fortunately, a variety of sensitive methods have become available for the identification and characterization of proteins separated by 2-DE, including Western immunoblotting, microsequencing by automated Edman degradation, amino acid compositional analysis, and, in particular, mass spectrometry. Readers interested in a more-detailed introduction to the technology of proteomics are referred to two recent books.[53,54]

Researchers have been quick to realize the potential of proteomics to characterize alterations in protein expression in heart disease and failure (reviewed in Reference 55). The results of these studies are providing new insights into the cellular mechanisms involved in cardiac dysfunction and are likely to lead to novel diagnostic markers and new therapeutic opportunities.

Recently, we have used the proteomic approach to explore changes in cardiac proteins in response to the chronic effects of alcohol.[57] In this study, the protein composition of hearts of rats fed ethanol for 6 weeks was compared with that of hearts of control rats not receiving alcohol in their diet. Of the more than 1000 cardiac proteins, which were separated by 2-DE, some 411 protein spots that could be detected on all the 2-D gel profiles were selected for analysis. Of these proteins, 10% were found to be altered in response to alcohol, with 7% being significantly increased in intensity while 3% were present at decreased intensity. Figure 3.3 shows a 2-D gel protein pattern in which several proteins differing significantly between control and alcohol-fed rats have been indicated, while Figure 3.4 shows an enlargement of the 29.9-kDa pI 6.7 region illustrating differences in one of these proteins (SSP 7319). In this study, some of the proteins showing significant differences between the two groups were identified by comparison to our human myocardial 2-DE protein database.[56] Among those proteins reduced in abundance were Heat Shock Proteins (HSP) 60 and 70. The significance of this finding is unclear at the moment, but consideration should be given to the fact that HSPs are important in cytosolic or mitochondrial protection, possibly implying ethanol-exposed heart may be more susceptible to cardioderangements. The intermediate filament protein desmin was also decreased, and this may have structural significance. Two isoforms of myosin light chain 2 were also decreased, while creatine kinase was increased. However, a considerable

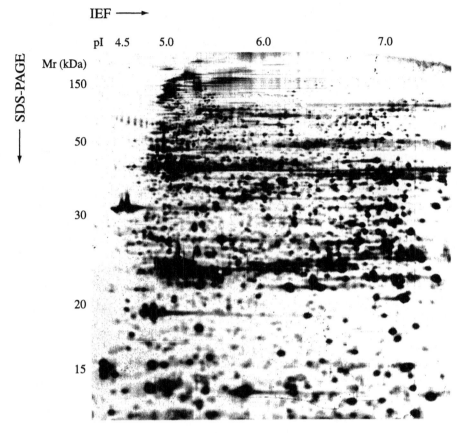

FIGURE 3.2
A typical 2-DE separation profile of total proteins (80 μg loading) of the rat heart visualized by silver staining. Approximately 1500 protein spots were detected on the original gel image. The scale at the top (first IEF dimension) indicates the isoelectric points (pI) of the separated proteins, while the scale at the left (second SDS-PAGE dimension) indicates their molecular weight (kDa). (From Patel, V.B. et al., *Electrophoresis*, 18, 2788, 1997. With permission.)

number of the proteins altered in response to alcohol remain uncharacterized. In addition, future work is planned to extend this proteomic approach to the investigation of alterations in cardiac proteins in biopsy specimens from cases of human alcoholic heart muscle disease.

Conclusion

Alcoholic heart muscle disease, also called alcoholic cardiomyopathy, is a consequence of chronic ethanol misuse. In particular, there is a relationship to the cumulative intake of ethanol rather than recent consumption. A variety

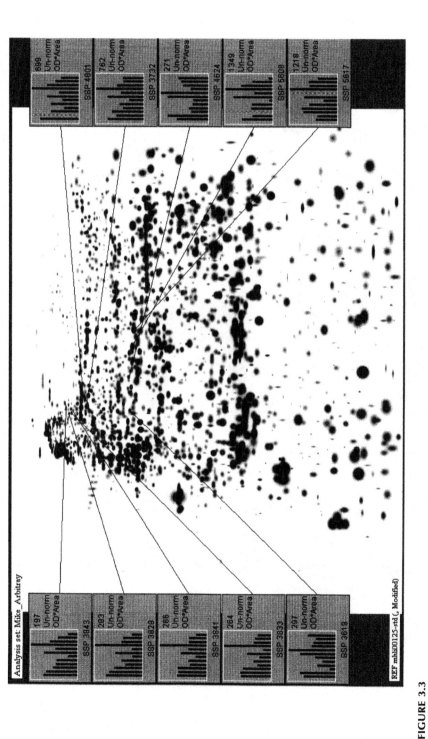

FIGURE 3.3

Computer database 2-DE master image for the study of changes in rat cardiac proteins in response to the chronic effects of alcohol. Several protein spots showing significant quantitative differences between control and alcohol-fed rats are indicated. The histograms on either side show the relative abundance of particular protein spots (indicated by SSP numbers) in six pairs of rats (control rat followed by the respective pair-fed alcohol-treated rat). (From Patel, V.B. et al., *Electrophoresis*, 18, 2788, 1997. With permission.)

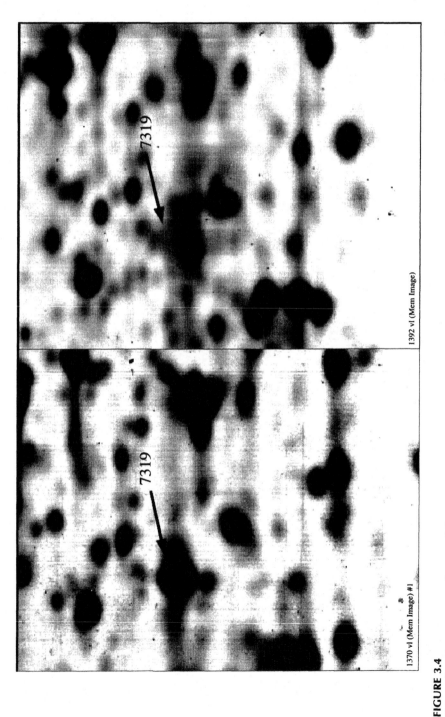

FIGURE 3.4

Enlarged computer images showing differences in spot SSP 7319 (molecular weight 29.9 kDa and pI 6.7), where the intensity of this protein is significantly reduced in the alcohol-fed rat. (From Patel, V.B. et al., *Electrophoresis*, 18, 2788, 1997. With permission.)

of biochemical lesions occur and appropriate animal models have facilitated studies into this disease. These models take into account the possible nutritional component of alcohol misuse. However, we can now conclude that malnutrition is not a causative factor in the pathogenesis of alcoholic cardiomyopathy and more discrete biochemical mechanisms occur, including the formation of acetaldehyde–protein adducts and changes in myocardial enzymatic activities. The application of proteomics has further shown that there are multiple derangements in a number of proteins including contractile, cytoskeletal, and regulatory proteins. Further studies are also needed to characterize whether similar proteomics changes occur in clinical samples.

References

1. Friedman, H.S., Cardiovascular effects of alcohol, *Recent Dev. Alcohol.*, 14, 135, 1998.
2. Urbano Marquez, A., Estruch, R., Navarro Lopez, F., Grau, J.M., Mont, L., and Rubin, E., The effects of alcoholism on skeletal and cardiac muscle, *N. Engl. J. Med.*, 320, 409, 1989.
3. Rubin, E. and Urbano Marquez, A., Clinical effects of alcohol on the cardiovascular system, in *Alcohol and the Cardiovascular System*, Zakhari, S. and Wassef, M., Eds., National Institutes of Health, Bethesda, 1996, 127.
4. Teragaki, M., Takeuchi, K., and Takeda, T., Clinical and histologic features of alcohol drinkers with congestive heart failure, *Am. Heart J.*, 125, 808, 1993.
5. Richardson, P.J. and Wodak, A., Alcohol-induced heart muscle disease, Symons, C., Evans, T., and Mitchell, A.G., Eds., Wright PSG, Bristol, 1983, 99.
6. Richardson, P.J., Wodak, A.D., Atkinson, L., Saunders, J.B., and Jewitt, D.E., Relation between alcohol intake, myocardial enzyme activity, and myocardial function in dilated cardiomyopathy, Evidence for the concept of alcohol induced heart muscle disease, *Br. Heart J.*, 56, 165, 1986.
7. Cerqueira, M.D., Harp, G.D., Ritchie, J.L., Stratton, J.R., and Walker, R.D., Rarity of preclinical alcoholic cardiomyopathy in chronic alcoholics less than 40 years of age, *Am. J. Cardiol.*, 67, 183, 1991.
8. Gillet, C., Juilliere, Y., Pirollet, P., Aubin, H. J., Thouvenin, A., Danchin, N., Cherrier, F., and Paille, F., Alcohol consumption and biological markers for alcoholism in idiopathic dilated cardiomyopathy: a case-controlled study, *Alcohol Alcohol.*, 27, 353, 1992.
9. Preedy, V.R., Why, H., Paice, A.G., Reilly, M.E., Ansell, H., Patel V.B., and Richardson, P.J., Protein synthesis in the heart *in vivo*, its measurement and patho-physiological alterations, *Int. J. Cardiol.*, 50, 95, 1995.
10. Preedy, V.R. and Richardson, P.J., Alcoholic cardiomyopathy: clinical and experimental pathological changes, *Herz*, 21, 241, 1996.
11. Patel, V.B., Why, H.J., Richardson, P.J., and Preedy, V.R., The effects of alcohol on the heart, *Adverse Drug React. Toxicol. Rev.*, 16, 15, 1997.
12. Preedy, V.R. and Richardson, P.J., Alcohol and the heart, in *Current Issues in Cardiovascular Therapy*, Elliott, H.L., Ed., Martin Dunitz, London, 1997, p. 83.

13. Richardson, P.J., Patel, V.B., and Preedy, V.R., Alcohol and the myocardium, *Novartis Found. Symp.*, 216, 35, 1998.
14. Agren, G. and Jakobsson, S.W., Validation of diagnoses on death certificates for male alcoholics in Stockholm, *Forensic Sci. Int.*, 33, 231, 1987.
15. Romelsjo, A., Karlsson, G., Henningsohn, L., and Jakobsson, S.W., The prevalence of alcohol-related mortality in both sexes: variation between indicators, Stockholm, 1987, *Am. J. Public Health*, 83, 838, 1993.
16. Lau, G., Natural disease and alcohol intoxication amongst drivers of motor vehicles in Singapore from 1989 to 1993: a study of 140 necropsies, *Ann. Acad. Med. Singapore*, 25, 516, 1996.
17. Ahmed, A.N., Elton, R.A., and Busuttil, A., Assessment of myocardial vasculature in chronic alcoholics without established cardiomyopathy, *Int. J. Legal. Med.*, 109, 167, 1996.
18. Vasiljevic, J.D., Kanjuh, V., Seferovic, P., and Olsen, E.G., Diagnostic endomyocardial biopsy findings in 160 consecutive patients: the Yugoslavian experience, *Am. J. Cardiovasc. Pathol.*, 3, 199, 1990.
19. Seferovic, P.M., Maksimovic, R., Ostojic, M., Stepanovic, S., Nikolic, J., Vasiljevic, J.D., Kanjuh, V., Seferovic, D., Simeunovic, S., Ristic, A. et al., Myocardial catecholamines in primary heart muscle disease: fact or fancy? *Eur. Heart J.*, 16 Suppl. O, 124, 1995.
20. La Vecchia, L.L., Bedogni, F., Bozzola, L., Bevilacqua, P., Ometto, R., and Vincenzi, M., Prediction of recovery after abstinence in alcoholic cardiomyopathy: role of hemodynamic and morphometric parameters, *Clin. Cardiol.*, 19, 45, 1996.
21. Sudarikova, Yu, Bakeeva, L.E., and Tsiplenkova, V.G., Ultrastructure of mitochondrial reticulum of human cardiomyocytes in alcohol cardiomyopathy, *Biochem. Mosc.*, 62, 989, 1997.
22. Preedy, V.R., Duane, P., and Peters, T.J., Biological effects of chronic ethanol consumption: a reappraisal of the Lieber-De Carli liquid-diet model with reference to skeletal muscle, *Alcohol Alcohol.*, 23, 151, 1988.
23. Preedy, V.R., McIntosh, A., Bonner, A.B., and Peters, T.J., Ethanol dosage regimens in studies of ethanol toxicity: influence of nutrition and surgical interventions, *Addict. Biol.*, 1, 255, 1996.
24. Burch, G.E., Colcolough, H.L., Harb, J.M., and Tsui, C.Y., The effect of ingestion of ethyl alcohol, wine and beer on the myocardium of mice, *Am. J. Cardiol.*, 27, 522, 1971.
25. Czarnecki, C.M., Schaffer, S.W., and Evanson, O.A., Ultrastructural features of ethanol-induced cardiomyopathy in turkey poults, *Comp. Biochem. Physiol. A.*, 82, 939, 1985.
26. Capasso, J.M., Li, P., Guideri, G., and Anversa, P., Left ventricular dysfunction induced by chronic alcohol ingestion in rats, *Am. J. Physiol.*, 261, H212, 1991.
27. Segel, L.D., Rendig, S.V., Choquet, Y., Chacko, K., Amsterdam, E.A., and Mason, D.T., Effects of chronic graded ethanol consumption on the metabolism, ultrastructure, and mechanical function of the rat heart, *Cardiovasc. Res.*, 9, 649, 1975.
28. Segel, L.D., The development of alcohol-induced cardiac dysfunction in the rat, *Alcohol Alcohol.*, 23, 391, 1988.
29. Preedy, V.R. and Peters, T.J., The acute and chronic effects of ethanol on cardiac muscle protein synthesis in the rat *in vivo*, *Alcohol*, 7, 97, 1990.
30. Morvai, V. and Ungvary, G., Effect of chronic exposure to alcohol on the circulation of rats of different ages, *Acta Physiol. Acad. Sci. Hung.*, 53, 433, 1979.

31. Jaatinen, P.I., Saukko, P., Sarviharju, M., Kiianmaa, K., and Hervonen, A., Effects of lifelong ethanol consumption on the ultrastructure and lipopigmentation of rat heart, *Alcohol Alcohol.*, 29, 269, 1994.

32. Brown, R.A., Savage, A.O., and Lloyd, T.C., Influence of age on the inotropic response to acute ethanol exposure in spontaneously hypertensive rats, *Hypertension*, 28, 872, 1996.

33. Worrall, S., de Jersey, J., Shanley, B.C., and Wilce, P.A., Detection of stable acetaldehyde-modified proteins in ethanol-fed rats, *Alcohol Alcohol.*, 26, 437, 1991.

34. Sotomayor, R.E. and Washington, M.C., Formation of etheno and oxoethyl adducts in liver DNA from rats exposed subchronically to urethane in drinking water and ethanol, *Cancer Lett.*, 100, 155, 1996.

35. Harcombe, A.A., Ramsay, L., Kenna, J.G., Koskinas, J., Why, H.J., Richardson P.J., Weissberg, P.L., and Alexander G.J., Circulating antibodies to cardiac protein-acetaldehyde adducts in alcoholic heart muscle disease, *Clin. Sci.*, 88, 263, 1995.

36. Worrall, S., de Jersey, J., Shanley, B. C., and Wilce, P. A., Antibodies to acetaldehyde-modified epitopes: an elevated immunoglobulin A response in alcoholics. *Eur. J. Clin. Invest.*, 21, 90, 1991.

37. Worrall, S., de Jersey, J., Wilce, P. A., Seppa, K., Hurme, L., and Sillanaukee, P., Relationship between alcohol intake and immunoglobulin a immunoreactivity with acetaldehyde-modified bovine serum albumin, *Alcohol. Clin. Exp. Res.*, 20, 836, 1996.

38. Xu, D., Thiele, G.M., Kearley, M.L., Haugen, M.D., Klassen, L.W., Sorrell, M.F., and Tuma, D.J., Epitope characterization of malondialdehyde-acetaldehyde adducts using an enzyme-linked immunosorbent assay, *Chem. Res Toxicol.*, 10, 978, 1997.

39. Dupont, I., Lucas, D., Clot, P., Menez, C., and Albano, E., Cytochrome P4502E1 inducibility and hydroxyethyl radical formation among alcoholics, *J. Hepatol.*, 28, 564, 1998.

40. Worrall, S., de Jersey, J., and Wilce, P.A., Comparison of the formation of proteins modified by direct and indirect metabolites of ethanol in the liver and blood of rats fed the Lieber-DeCarli diet, *Alcohol Alcohol.*, 35, 2000.

41. Deitrich, R.A., Tissue and subcellular distribution of mammalian aldehyde-oxydizing capacity, *Biochem. Pharmacol.*, 15, 1911, 1966.

42. Nagasawa, H.T. and Alexander, C.S., Ethanol metabolism by the rat heart and alcohol dehydrogenase activity, *Can. J. Biochem.*, 54, 539, 1976.

43. Holmes, R.S., Courtney, Y.R., and VandeBerg, J.L., Alcohol dehydrogenase isozymes in baboons: tissue distribution, catalytic properties, and variant phenotypes in liver, kidney, stomach, and testis, *Alcohol. Clin. Exp. Res.*, 10, 623, 1986.

44. Julia, P., Farres, J., and Pares, X., Characterization of three isoenzymes of rat alcohol dehydrogenase. Tissue distribution and physical and enzymatic properties, *Eur. J. Biochem.*, 162, 179, 1987.

45. Felder, M.R., Watson, G., Huff, M.O., and Ceci, J.D., Mechanism of induction of mouse kidney alcohol dehydrogenase by androgen. Androgen-induced stimulation of transcription of the Adh-1 gene, *J. Biol Chem.*, 263, 14531, 1988.

46. Jukkola, A. and Niemela, O., Covalent binding of acetaldehyde to type III collagen, *Biochem. Biophys. Res. Commun.*, 159, 163, 1989.

47. Niemela, O., Acetaldehyde adducts of proteins: diagnostic and pathogenic implications in diseases caused by excessive alcohol consumption, *Scand. J. Clin. Lab. Invest. Suppl.*, 213, 45, 1993.
48. Hill, G.E., Miller, J.A., Baxter, B.T., Klassen, L.W., Duryee, M.J., Tuma, D.J., and Thiele, G.M., Association of malondialdehyde-acetaldehyde (MAA) adducted proteins with atherosclerotic-induced vascular inflammatory injury, *Atherosclerosis*, 141, 107, 1998.
49. Gvozdjakova, A., Kuznetsov, A.V., Kucharska, J., Miklovicova, E., and Gvozdjak, J., The functional state of the creatine kinase system of myocardial mitochondria in alcoholic cardiomyopathy, *Cor. Vasa.*, 33, 343, 1991.
50. Klatsky, A.L., Alcohol, coronary disease, and hypertension, *Annu. Rev. Med.*, 47, 149, 1996.
51. Puddey, I.B., Beilin, L.J., and Rakic, V., Alcohol, hypertension and the cardiovascular system: a critical appraisal, *Addict. Biol.*, 2, 159, 1997.
52. Wasinger, V.C., Cordwell, S.J., Cerpa-Poljak, A., Yan, J.X., Gooley, A.A., Wilkins, M.R., Duncan, M.W., Harris, R., Williams, K.L., Humphery, Smith, I., Progress with gene-product mapping of the Mollicutes: mycoplasma genitalium, *Electrophoresis*, 16, 1090, 1995.
53. Wilkins, M.R., Williams, K.L., Appel, R.D., and Hochstrasser, D.F., *Proteome Research: New Frontiers in Functional Genomics*, Springer-Verlag, Heidelberg, 1997.
54. Rabilloud, T., *Proteome Research: Two-Dimensional Gel Electrophoresis and Identification Methods*, Springer-Verlag, Heidelberg, 2000.
55. Dunn, M.J., Studying heart disease using the proteomic approach, *Drug Discovery Today*, 5, 76, 2000.
56. Evans, G., Wheeler, C.H., Corbett, J.M., and Dunn, M.J., Construction of HSC-2DPAGE: a two-dimensional gel electrophoresis database of heart proteins, *Electrophoresis*, 18, 471, 1997.
57. Patel, V.B., Corbett, J.M., Dunn, M.J., Winrow, V.R., Portmann, B., Richardson, P.J., and Preedy V.R., Protein profiling in cardiac tissue in response to the chronic effects of alcohol, *Electrophoresis*, 18, 2788, 1997.

4

Age, Gender, and Body Composition: Implications for Alcohol Research in Older Persons

Becky T. Davies

CONTENTS

Introduction

Provocative titles such as "Aging and Ethanol Metabolism,"[1] "Age, Drinking Habits and the Effects of Alcohol,"[2] and "Alcohol Pharmacodynamics in Young-Elderly Adults Contrasted with Young and Middle-Aged Subjects,"[3] suggest that researchers have sought a thorough understanding of the effects of age on an individual's physiological response to alcohol. Closer inspection, however, reveals that none of these studies included females.

In fact, with the exception of two very recent studies,[4,5] a search of published alcohol research reveals only a few experimental trials designed specifically to address the physiological consequences of alcohol consumption by older women.[6-9]

From an epidemiological standpoint, researchers have consistently found that women suffer from alcohol-induced liver disease,[10] brain damage,[11] and alcoholic cardiomyopathy[12] at what appears to be a lesser lifetime exposure to alcohol compared with men suffering from these diseases. Recent experimental studies have also found that alcohol increases the level of circulating estradiol in postmenopausal women receiving estrogen replacement therapy,[6] an effect linked to disrupted cholesterol levels and a higher incidence of breast cancer.

These findings suggest the need for more extensive investigations of the effects of alcohol on females in general, and older females in particular. Yet, females and older persons are routinely excluded from alcohol studies. The higher blood alcohol concentrations (BACs) frequently observed in these subject groups introduce a degree of variability in the data that researchers have found both annoying and difficult to reconcile.

The relatively small number of studies that purport to have tested "older" males have found an association between a subject's age and peak blood alcohol concentration.[1,3,13] However, such investigations suffer from two shortcomings. The most obvious problem with these studies is their inclusion of very few "older" males, many of whom are not beyond 60 years of age. The less obvious weakness, which is present in virtually all studies involving older persons, is a methodological one that is the subject of this chapter.

Estimation of Peak Blood Alcohol Concentration

Widmark's[14] investigations concerning ethanol metabolism were conducted to gain a better understanding of alcohol pharmacokinetics (the distribution of alcohol within the body, as well as the elimination of alcohol from the body). Widmark's original study sample consisted of only 20 males and 10 females. The information gathered on these 30 subjects was used to formulate an equation by which to describe the relationship between the total amount of alcohol ingested, the concentration of alcohol in the blood at a given time, and body weight.

Widmark established the factor "r" to indicate the fraction of the body mass into which alcohol is distributed.[15] Gender differences in the values that could be assigned to r were noted such that males had an average $r = 0.68$ and females had an average $r = 0.55$. The general impressions regarding the distribution of alcohol in the body gained from this small sample of individuals remains fundamental to forensic alcohol analyses and provides the basic formula (known as the "Widmark equation") by which to predict the blood alcohol concentation (BAC) that will likely be attained by a given individual.[16,17]

Body Composition Factors and BAC

A number of factors in an individual person's physiological profile (e.g., age, gender, body size, drinking history) have since been investigated by researchers interested in more accurately estimating the amount of alcohol a person must consume to reach a certain BAC. Since Widmark's original work in 1932, there have been several revisions of the equations used by researchers to predict blood alcohol concentration.

Alcohol readily diffuses into the body's water compartment.[18] Thus, Widmark's *r* has been equated with the amount of water in the body.[15] Watson et al.[19] updated Widmark's work and provided equations for expressing the relationship between the amount of alcohol ingested and BAC in terms of a person's total body water (TBW). The Watson "Alcohol:Total Body Water" equation is more complex than that originally formulated by Widmark, in that it emphasizes not only body weight and gender as important determinants of a person's BAC, but age as well. Although previous work by Watson and colleagues[20] specifies that age is not an important factor in determining the TBW for females, this important point is frequently overlooked by alcohol researchers when interpreting the effects of gender, age, and TBW on resultant BACs in groups of subjects.

Two very general (albeit well-accepted) statements have been generated through years of research based on the work of Widmark, Watson, and others. First, females typically reach higher BACs than males for a given dose of alcohol because the female's body contains proportionately more body fat and less body water.[21-27] Second, higher peak BACs are attained by older males compared with their younger counterparts because of the relative decrease in body water consequent to aging.[1,2,13] These gender- and age-related differences in body water are readily invoked by alcohol researchers who are anxious to explain how two individuals of equal body weight can reach widely discrepant BACs following consumption of a given amount of alcohol.[1,13,28,29]

Nevertheless, implicit within these generalizations lie naive assumptions about the importance of the "relative" amounts (or *percentages*) of body fat and body water that constitute body weight. Estimation of a person's percentage of body fat (by means of hydrodensitometry[30] or measures of skinfold thickness[31]) was once the only reliable means of determining a person's body water without resorting to more costly radioisotope dilution methods. Fat-free body mass contains a relatively constant amount of water (about 72 to 73%),[32] and there is an inverse relationship between body fat and body water.[28,31,33] Thus, body water can be estimated by means of a simple calculation when a person's body weight and percent body fat are known.

Aside from problems with the accuracy of these various estimates of body water for subgroups of the population, a more serious problem has arisen as alcohol researchers have embraced these concepts and used them to describe the impact of various body composition factors on BAC. The term *body water content* has been adopted as a vague term for the amount of water in a person's body. Under the auspices of body water content, body water as a percentage of body weight has been used interchangeably with TBW volume so frequently that many researchers fail to note the difference. (For an excellent example of this problem, see Marshall et al.,[34] and compare the usages of TBW in their Figures 2 and 3.)

However, the correspondence between body water expressed as a percentage of body weight and total body water volume in liters is not reliable. Certainly, this relationship becomes much more complex and variable when factors such as age, gender, and obesity are taken into consideration. The failure to appreciate this subtle distinction is likely responsible for a great deal of the confusion regarding the variability in peak BACs that are frequently observed in "diverse" subject groups (i.e., males and females, older persons and younger persons, obese persons and lean individuals). In an effort to reconcile seemingly conflicting research results, investigators have been more inclined to cite the obvious differences among subject groups in percentages of body fat and/or body water rather than search for more heuristically meaningful explanations.

Recent Research Findings

The following data are part of a larger data set comparing body composition factors and BACs in males and females in three age groups (Davies, unpublished results). Portions of these data have been analyzed and published previously.[4] For the sake of clarity, only the data pertaining to the younger (21 to 25 years old) and older ($\geq$ age 60 years) age groups are presented here.

For a complete description of the methods used, see Davies and Bowen.[4] Briefly, various dimensions of body composition were measured in young males ($n = 20$), young females ($n = 20$), older males ($n = 16$), and older females ($n = 16$). These data are presented in Tables 4.1 and 4.2.

Regardless of age, gender, or body composition, each subject in the study received an equal amount of alcohol (40 ml of 95% ethanol, equivalent to 30 g alcohol). The peak BAC for each person was then determined. In effect, since an equal amount of alcohol was administered to each subject, each person's body composition factors (body weight, total body water, age, gender, etc.) were allowed to determine the amount of alcohol received by that person.

Thus, the grams of alcohol per kilogram of body weight, as well as the grams of alcohol per liter of total body water, were *dependent variables* in this study. This method of administering alcohol produced some interesting results. See Tables 4.1 and 4.2 for the average grams per kilogram and grams per liter amounts of alcohol received by each group of subjects.

TABLE 4.1

Comparison of Body Composition Factors and BACs in Females

Comparison Measure x̄ (± S.D.)	Younger Females	Older Females
Age	21.8 (1.1)	68.9 (7.9)
Height (cm)	163.6 (7.4)	162.6 (4.0)
Weight (kg)	60.8 (10.7)	70.7 (13.8)
% body fat	29.9 (6.5)	37.5 (6.7)
TBW volume (l)	30.8 (3.0)	31.2 (3.1)
% body water	51.3 (4.6)	45.0 (4.8)
g/kg dose of alcohol	0.506 (0.081)	0.440 (0.088)
g/l dose of alcohol	0.983 (0.095)	0.970 (0.093)
BAC (g/dl)	0.0811 (0.012)	0.0975 (0.017)

TABLE 4.2

Comparison of Body Composition Factors and BACs in Males

Comparison Measure x̄ (+ S.D.)	Younger Males	Older Males
Age	21.9 (1.1)	67.0 (4.5)
Height (cm)	179.6 (5.7)	177.0 (5.1)
Weight (kg)	80.8 (11.3)	89.5 (12.4)
% body fat	18.8 (5.1)	29.8 (4.9)
TBW volume (l)	47.0 (5.6)	44.8 (3.3)
% body water	58.3 (3.6)	50.6 (3.5)
g/kg dose of alcohol	0.378 (0.054)	0.341 (.0046)
g/l dose of alcohol	0.646 (0.076)	0.672 (0.050)
BAC (g/dl)	0.0581 (0.013)	0.0600 (0.007)

Younger and Older Females

Investigators have come to anticipate the higher BACs that are frequently observed in females and older persons when they are administered doses of alcohol according to their body weight. However, higher BACs were reached by the older females in this study (x̄ BAC = 0.0975 compared with 0.0811 for younger females) in spite of the fact that they received a slightly smaller dose of alcohol in terms of body weight (0.440 g/kg compared with 0.506).

Furthermore, higher BACs were obtained for the older females even though they received a slightly smaller dose of alcohol in terms of TBW volume (0.970 g/l compared with 0.983 g/l for the younger females). Although body water constituted a smaller *percentage* of the body weight in the older females (x̄ = 45% compared with 51% in the younger females), the TBW volume of the older females was equivalent to that of the younger females (x̄ TBW = 31.2 and 30.8 l, respectively).

Younger and Older Males

In contrast to the data collected on the females, the data obtained on the males did not demonstrate any appreciable differences in BACs as a function of age. Thus, the BACs for the older and younger males were comparable ($\bar{x}$ BAC = 0.0600 and 0.0581, respectively) when alcohol was not administered according to body weight.

Although the older males had a much smaller percentage of body water, this was accompanied by only a slightly smaller TBW volume. The older males had an average of 50.6% body water compared with 58.3% in the younger males. Yet, the TBW volumes differed only slightly ($\bar{x}$ = 44.8 l TBW in the older male compared with $\bar{x}$ = 47.0 l TBW in the younger males). Thus, the slightly higher dose of alcohol received by older males in terms of TBW volume (0.672 g/l in the older male compared with 0.646 g/l in the younger male) was matched by an equally slight difference in BACs.

Age and Gender Comparisons

The data collected on these subjects are also represented graphically in Figures 4.1 through 4.3. Figure 4.1 shows the relationship between body water expressed as a percentage of body weight and the TBW for all 72 subjects in this data set. There is a slight *positive* correlation between percent body water and TBW such that a higher percentage of body water is associated with a larger TBW volume, as would be expected.

Figure 4.2 presents the identical data set as that represented in Figure 4.1, but with each subject group depicted separately. Separate trend lines have also been added for males and females. When the same data are presented in this way, the trends in the data are in the opposite direction. Thus, there is a slight *negative* correlation between percent body water and TBW for the males as a group, and a stronger *negative* correlation between percent body water and TBW for the females as a group. When each gender is considered separately, a highly illogical situation arises such that a *smaller percentage* of body water is associated with a *larger volume* of TBW.

The apparent reversal of the trend in the data from Figure 4.1 to Figure 4.2 is also known as "Simpson's paradox." The different interpretations of the data gleaned from the two figures are a direct consequence of incorrectly combining the results from two groups with different (i.e., offset) ranges of data. In addition, the wide range of percent body water values for both males and females presents another problem. Alcohol researchers frequently refer to the "average" percent body water values for males (55%) and females (45%) to account for discrepant BAC results. However, the results presented here seriously challenge this notion as a scientifically meaningful explanation for these differences.

A similar problem arises with the data in Figure 4.2 when one tries to discern the percent body water for an older subject vs. a younger subject within gender. For example, both older and younger females have an average of 31 liters of TBW. However, this same 31 liters represents anywhere from 42% of

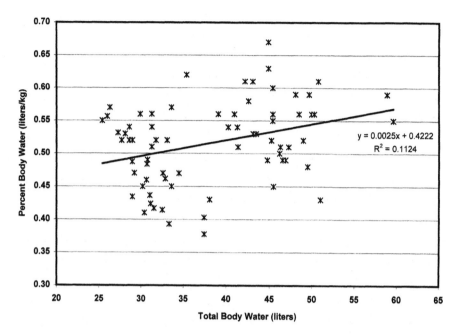

FIGURE 4.1

Scatter plot of percent body water (liters of water/kilogram of body weight) and total body water volume (in liters) for all 72 subjects.

the body weight in one of the older females to 57% of the body weight in one of the younger females. Do older females, then, have "less" body water than younger females?

The data for the males in this data set are equally ambiguous. For the males in this study, 45 liters of TBW can represent as little as 45% of the body weight in an older male, or as much as 68% of the body weight in a younger male. Thus, statements about the "smaller amount" of body water in older persons relative to younger persons become virtually meaningless in terms of a measurable TBW volume.

TBW Volume and BAC

The relationship between TBW volume and BAC for all 72 subjects is presented in Figure 4.3. Unlike the data in Figure 4.2, the data in Figure 4.3 present a consistent pattern of results for all four groups of subjects. That is, a strong negative correlation exists between TBW and BAC, such that a smaller volume of TBW is associated with a higher concentration of alcohol in the body, as would be expected. Thus, regardless of age, gender, or percent body water, knowledge of a person's TBW would be helpful in estimating the BAC that person might reach following consumption of 30 g of alcohol.

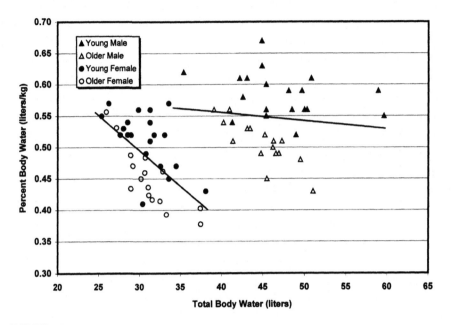

FIGURE 4.2
Scatter plot of the identical data presented in Figure 4.1, with each subject group depicted separately. The trend lines indicate the relationship between percent body water and TBW for males and females considered separately.

The data presented in Figure 4.3 also clearly depict the contrast in results that were obtained for the older males and older females. All but one of the data points for the older females in Figure 4.3 lie at or above the trend line. This pattern of results indicates that, for an equivalent amount of TBW, older females reach a higher BAC than younger females. In contrast, the data obtained on the males in this study failed to demonstrate any appreciable difference in BACs between younger and older males at near-equivalent TBW volumes.

Age-Related Gender Differences

General statements about the "smaller amount of body water" present in females compared with males, and older persons compared with younger individuals, have given investigators the false impression that the effects of age on a person's physiological response to alcohol are understood. Apparently, it has been assumed that the decrease in percent body water that occurs with age is accompanied by an equally precipitous drop in total body water

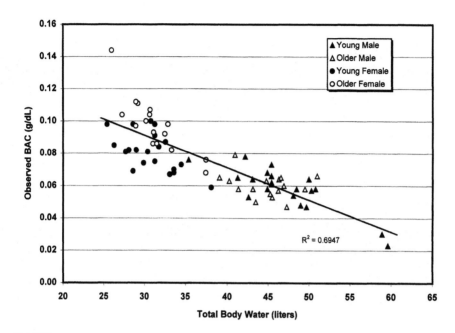

FIGURE 4.3

Scatter plot of observed BACs and TBW volume for each subject by subject group. The trend line indicates the relationship between observed BAC and TBW for all 72 subjects.

volume in both males and females.[35-38] The results presented here demonstrate that this is not necessarily the case.

Moreover, recent body composition studies indicate that these age-related changes may be different for men and women.[39,40] Older males experience a more pronounced decrease in lean body mass associated with increased adipose tissue.[41] In contrast, women lose less muscle mass as they age.[39] There is also evidence to suggest that the hydration of fat-free mass (muscle tissue) increases in older females.[42] The net result is that women retain more of their body water volume as they age in comparison to men.[39-42] The impact of these differential changes in body composition has not been fully recognized in alcohol research.

Methodological and Conceptual Issues

Historically, the majority of alcohol research has been conducted on younger males as investigators have attempted to restrict the variability in the peak BACs that are obtained. Thus, research on young males of similar body size provides the bulk of our knowledge of the physiological effects of alcohol ingestion. This practice has left researchers in the unfortunate position of treating the wealth of data that has been collected on the younger male as the "gold standard" against which the data obtained on other subject groups (i.e., females and older persons) must be compared.

Fundamental to this research has been the practice of administering alcohol according to body weight. This practice has continued in spite of evidence to suggest that weight-adjusted doses of alcohol can result in highly variable BACs, even in relatively homogeneous populations.[28,29,33] Yet, investigators persist in adhering to this procedure, even when administering alcohol to more heterogeneous subgroups.[3,13,16,17,22] As a remedy for the ever-increasing variability in BACs that can result from using this approach, researchers have attempted to adjust the dose of alcohol by the average percent body water for a given group of subjects.[21,24-26,28,33,34,37]

Although such adjustments in alcohol doses often lessen the variability in the BACs that are obtained, they do nothing toward furthering our understanding of the disposition of alcohol in the body. Rather than providing a remedy to the problem, these methods only add to the confusion. Thus, investigators continue to employ an unreliable method (dosing by body weight) and attempt to correct it by applying misbegotten notions about the "amount" of body water in males and females, and older persons vs. younger persons.

Volume of Distribution for Ethanol

There is little question that, upon ingestion, alcohol distributes into the body's water compartment.[18,42-44] Indeed, TBW volume may provide the best estimate of the volume of distribution for ethanol in the body.[45-47] Thus, body water governs the blood and tissue concentrations of alcohol.[14,15] An estimate of body water has therefore been proposed as the best indicator of the biological impact of consuming a given amount of alcohol.[46-48]

It is for this reason that health professionals have cautioned both women and older persons about the medical consequences of ingesting alcoholic beverages.[35,36,48] Several researchers have also suggested that alcohol consumption measures be adjusted to reflect the age- and gender-related differences in percent body water.[37,38,48,49] However, as has been seen, percent body water is an unreliable metric, which can produce false and/or misleading results.

Implications for Further Research

The Davies and Bowen[4] and Lucey et al.[5] studies of the effects of alcohol in older females reached the same conclusion: The higher BACs attained by older females cannot be fully accounted for by body water volume. This result can have important implications, both methodological and conceptual, for future research. The biological impact of alcohol consumption in older females should be explored both epidemiologically and experimentally in the reference population (i.e., older females).

Likewise, the results presented here for the older male suggest that additional studies are warranted to establish the physiological impact of alcohol in this population. Previous studies comparing older and younger males may have been compromised by a serious methodological problem. That is, the higher BACs observed in older males are an artifact of dosing subjects by body weight. As such, these results contribute little toward our understanding of the disposition of alcohol in the body of older males.

In light of the aging of our population, the differential effects of gender, age, and body composition factors on the physiological consequences of alcohol consumption by older persons need further investigation. In particular, there have been suggestions that (1) age decreases the volume of distribution for ethanol in the body[2,13,37,48] and (2) chronic consumption of alcohol increases the volume of distribution for ethanol.[50-53] If indeed distinct (measurable) physiological changes associated with these observations exist, they must be addressed without reliance upon vague generalizations concerning the percentages of body fat and body water present in men vs. women,[24-26,34,54] or older persons vs. younger persons.[1,2,37] Only with a more consistent and precise understanding of the distribution of alcohol in older males and females will researchers be in a position to address more difficult issues, such as the recent suggestion that age may affect the severity and complications of alcohol withdrawal.[55]

References

1. Vestal, R.E., McGuire, E.A., Tobin, J.D., Andres, R., Norris, A.H., and Mezey, E., Aging and ethanol metabolism, *Clin. Pharmacol. Ther.*, 21, 343, 1977.
2. Vogel-Sprott, M. and Barrett, P., Age, drinking habits and the effects of alcohol, *J. Stud. Alcohol*, 45, 517, 1984.
3. Tupler, L.A., Hege, S., and Ellinwood, E.H., Alcohol pharmacodynamics in young-elderly adults contrasted with young and middle-aged subjects, *Psychopharmacology*, 118, 460, 1995.
4. Davies, B.T. and Bowen, C.K., Total body water and peak alcohol concentration: a comparative study of young, middle-age, and older females, *Alcohol. Clin. Exp. Res.*, 23, 969, 1999.
5. Lucey, M.R., Hill, E.M., Young, J.P., Demo-Dananberg, L., and Beresford, T.P., The influences of age and gender on blood ethanol concentrations in healthy humans, *J. Stud. Alcohol.*, 60, 103, 1999.
6. Ginsburg, E.S., Walsh, B.W., Shea, B.F., Gao, X., Gleason, R.E., and Barbieri, R.L., The effects of ethanol on the clearance of estradiol in postmenopausal women, *Fertil. Steril.*, 63, 1227, 1995.

7. Mendelson, J.H., Mello, N.K., Ellingboe, J., and Bavli, S., Alcohol effects on plasma luteinizing hormone levels in postmenopausal women, *Pharmacol. Biochem. Behav.*, 22, 233, 1985.

8. Stott, D.J., Dutton, M., Murray, G.D., Williams, B.O., and McInnes, G.T., Hemodynamic effects of a single moderate dose of alcohol in elderly subjects, *J. Stud. Alcohol.*, 52, 377, 1991.

9. Valimaki, M., Pelkonen, R., and Ylikahri, R., Acute ethanol intoxication does not influence gonadotropin secretion in postmenopausal women, *Alcohol Alcohol.*, 22, 143, 1987.

10. Becker, U., Deis, A., Sorensen, T.I.A., Gronbaek, M., Borch-Johnsen, K., Muller, C.F., Schnohr, P., and Jensen, G., Prediction of risk of liver disease by alcohol intake, sex, and age: a prospective population study, *Hepatology*, 23, 1025, 1996.

11. Mann, K., Batra, A., Gunthner, A., and Schroth, G., Do women develop alcoholic brain damage more readily than men? *Alcohol. Clin. Exp. Res.*, 16, 1052, 1992.

12. Urbano-Marquez, A., Estruch, R., Fernandez-Sola, J., Nicolas, J.M., Pare, J.C., and Rubin, E., The greater risk of alcoholic cardiomyopathy and myopathy in women compared with men, *JAMA*, 274, 149, 1995.

13. Jones, A.W. and Neri, A., Age-related differences in blood ethanol parameters and subjective feelings of intoxication in healthy men, *Alcohol Alcohol.*, 20, 45, 1985.

14. Widmark, E.M.P., *Die theoretischen Grundlagen und die praktische Verwendbarkeit der gerichlich-medizinischen Alkoholbestimmung*, Urban & Schwarzenberg, Berlin, 1932.

15. Baselt, R.C. and Danhof, I.E., Disposition of alcohol in man, in *Medicolegal Aspects of Alcohol Determination in Biological Specimens*, Garriott, J.C., Ed., PSG Publishing, Littleton, MS, 1988, 55–73.

16. Jones, A.W. and Jonsson, K.A., Between-subject and within-subject variations in the pharmacokinetics of ethanol, *Br. J. Clin. Pharmacol.*, 37, 427, 1994.

17. Jones, A.W. and Andersson, L., Influence of age, gender, and blood-alcohol concentration on the disappearance rate of alcohol from blood in drinking drivers, *J. Forensic Sci.*, 41, 922, 1996.

18. Harger, R.M. and Hulpieu, H.R., The pharmacology of alcohol, in *Alcoholism*, Thompson, G.N., Ed., Charles C. Thomas Publishers, Springfield, 1956, 103–232.

19. Watson, P.E., Watson, I.D., and Batt, R.D., Prediction of blood alcohol concentrations in human subjects: updating the Widmark equation, *J. Stud. Alcohol*, 42, 547, 1981.

20. Watson, P.E., Watson, I.D., and Batt, R.D., Total body water volumes for adult males and females estimated from simple anthropometric measurements, *Am. J. Clin. Nutr.*, 33, 27, 1980.

21. Church, M.W., Abel, E.L., Dintcheff, B.A., and Matyjasik, C., Maternal age and blood alcohol concentration in the pregnant Long-Evans rat, *J. Pharmacol. Exp. Ther.*, 253, 192, 1990.

22. Dubowski, K.M., Human pharmacokinetics of ethanol. I. Peak blood concentrations and elimination in male and female subjects, *Alcohol Tech. Rep.*, 5, 55, 1976.

23. Gearhart, J.G., Beebe, D.K., Milhorn, H.T., and Meeks, G.R., Alcoholism in women, *Am. Fam. Physician*, 44, 907, 1991.

24. Goist, K.C. and Sutker, P.B., Acute alcohol intoxication and body composition in women and men, *Pharmacol. Biochem. Behav.*, 22, 811, 1985.

25. Savoie, T.M., Emory, E.K., and Moody-Thomas, S., Acute alcohol intoxication in socially drinking female and male offspring of alcoholic fathers, *J. Stud. Alcohol*, 49, 430, 1988.

26. Sutker, P.B., Tabakoff, B., Goist, K.C., Jr., and Randall, C.L., Acute alcohol intoxication, mood states and alcohol metabolism in women and men, *Pharmacol. Biochem. Behav.*, 18(Suppl. 1), 349, 1983.

27. York, J.L., Body water content, ethanol pharmacokinetics, and the responsiveness to ethanol in young and old rats, *Dev. Pharmacol. Ther.*, 4, 106, 1982.

28. Devgun, M.S. and Dunbar, J.A., Alcohol consumption, blood alcohol level and the relevance of body weight in experimental design and analysis, *J. Stud. Alcohol.*, 51, 24, 1990.

29. O'Neill, B., Williams, A.F., and Dubowski, K.M., Variability in blood alcohol concentrations: implications for estimating individual results, *J. Stud. Alcohol.*, 44, 222, 1983.

30. Behnke, A.R., Feen, B.G., and Welham, W.C., Specific gravity of healthy men, *JAMA*, 118, 495, 1942.

31. Durnin, J.V.G.A. and Womersley, J., Body fat assessed from total body density and its estimation from skinfold thickness, *Br. J. Nutr.*, 32, 77, 1974.

32. Pace, N. and Rathburn, E.N., Studies on body composition. III. The body water and chemically combined nitrogen content in relation to fat content, *J. Biol. Chem.*, 158, 685, 1945.

33. Radlow, R. and Hurst, P.M., Temporal relations between blood alcohol concentration and alcohol effect: an experiment with human subjects, *Psychopharmacology*, 85, 260, 1985.

34. Marshall, A.W., Kingstone, D., Boss, M., and Morgan, M.Y., Ethanol elimination in males and females: relationship to menstrual cycle and body composition, *Hepatology*, 3, 701, 1983.

35. Scott, R.B., Alcohol effects in the elderly, *Comp. Ther.*, 15, 8, 1989.

36. Fink, A., Hays, R.D., Moore, A.A., and Beck, J.C., Alcohol-related problems in older persons: determinants, consequences, and screening, *Arch. Intern. Med.*, 156, 1150, 1996.

37. Dufour, M.C., Archer, L., and Gordis, E., Alcohol and the elderly, *Clin. Geriatr. Med.*, 8, 127, 1992.

38. Gambert, S.R., Alcohol abuse: medical effects of heavy drinking in late life, *Geriatrics*, 52, 30, 1997.

39. Going, S., Williams, D., and Lohman, T., Aging and body composition: biological changes and methodological issues, *Exercise Sports Sci. Rev.*, 23, 411, 1995.

40. Williams, D.P., Going, S.B., Milliken, L.A., Hall, M.C., and Lohman, T.G., Practical techniques for assessing body composition in middle-aged and older adults, *Med. Sci. Sports Exercise*, 27, 776, 1995.

41. Hewitt, M.J., Going, S.B., Williams, D.P., and Lohman, T.G., Hydration of the fat-free body mass in children and adults: implications for body composition assessment, *Am. J. Physiol.* 265 (*Endocrinol. Metab.*), 28, E88, 1993.

42. Endres, H.G.E. and Gruner, O., Comparison of D_2O and ethanol dilutions in total body water measurements in humans, *Clin. Invest.*, 72, 830, 1994.

43. Loeppky, J.A., Myhre, L.G., Venters, M.D., and Luft, U.C., Total body water and lean body mass estimated by ethanol dilution, *J. Appl. Physiol.*, 42, 803, 1977.

44. Tzamaloukas, A.H., Jackson, J.E., Gallegos, J.C., Long, D.A., and McLane, M.M., Distribution volume of ethanol as a measure of body water, *Miner. Electrolyte Metab.*, 11, 123, 1985.

45. Bosron, W.F., Ehrig, T., and Li, T.K., Genetic factors in alcohol metabolism and alcoholism, *Semin. Liver Dis.*, 13, 126, 1993.
46. York, J.L. and Hirsch, J.A., Application of bioelectrical impedance methodology and prediction equations to determine the volume of distribution for ethanol, *Alcohol*, 12, 553, 1995.
47. York, J.L. and Hirsch, J.A., Association between blood pressure and lifetime drinking patterns in moderate drinkers, *J. Stud. Alcohol.*, 58, 480, 1997.
48. Mirand, A.L. and Welte, J., Total body water adjustment of mean alcohol intakes, *J. Subst. Abuse*, 6, 419, 1994.
49. York, J.L. and Welte, J.W., Gender comparisons of alcohol consumption in alcoholic and nonalcoholic populations, *J. Stud. Alcohol.*, 55, 750, 1994.
50. York, J.L. and Pendergast, D.E., Body composition in detoxified alcoholics, *Alcohol. Clin. Exp. Res.*, 14, 180, 1990.
51. York, J.L., Progression of alcohol consumption across the drinking career in alcoholics and social drinkers, *J. Stud. Alcohol.*, 56, 328, 1995.
52. Holtzman, J.L., Gebhard, R.L., Eckfeldt, J.H., Mottonen, L.R., Finley, D.K., and Eshelman, F.N., The effects of several weeks of ethanol consumption on ethanol kinetics in normal men and women, *Clin. Pharmacol. Ther.*, 38, 157, 1985.
53. Whitfield, J.B. and Martin, N.G., Alcohol consumption and alcohol pharmacokinetics: interactions within the normal population, *Alcohol. Clin. Exp. Res.*, 18, 238, 1994.
54. Cowan, J.M., Weathermon, A., McCutcheon, J.R., and Oliver, R.D., Determination of volume of distribution for ethanol in male and female subjects, *J. Anal. Toxicol.*, 20, 287, 1996.
55. Kraemer, K.L., Mayo-Smith, M.F., and Calkins, D.R., Impact of age on the severity, course, and complications of alcohol withdrawal, *Arch. Intern. Med.*, 157, 2234, 1997.

5

Presentation and Rehabilitation of Elderly People with Alcohol-Related Problems

John Dickson Mulinga

CONTENTS

Introduction

Elderly people, that is, those aged 65 years and over, in general have physiological, biological, psychological, and socioeconomic changes that influence the way in which they present with clinical problems.[1,2] In turn, society tends to adopt an attitude that denies the existence of certain problems in elderly people, or, if acknowledged, the attitude is a laissez faire one. Alcohol and substance misuse in elderly people typifies this situation, with poor recognition of alcohol-related problems and subsequent poor efforts at rehabilitation.[2,3] Improving this situation will demand a better understanding not only of the relationship between age-related changes and alcohol-related problems in this age group, but also how best to offer treatment and rehabilitation to those affected. This, in turn, will depend on well-conducted age-specific research in this area. In this chapter, alcohol-related problems will be taken to equate to *alcohol abuse* or *harmful use* in DSM-IV and ICD-10 criteria, respectively, and alcohol dependence in both the above criteria. The rest of the chapter will discuss some aspects of the clinical presentation of elderly people with alcohol-related problems, especially those that differ significantly from those in younger alcohol abusers, as well as their rehabilitation. An illustrative case history will be discussed at the end. Discussion of individual complications or presentations is not intended.

Clinical Presentation

The majority of elderly people who drink alcohol do so without any problems whatsoever and may even benefit.[4,5] These are the low-risk or social drinkers. In common with the classification used in younger people, a proportion of the elderly population drink more than the recommended *safe* limit (*low-risk*) of *21 to 50* units of alcohol for men and *14 to 35* units per week for women. These are said to be in the *increasing risk* group. A further proportion will drink more than these limits, placing themselves in the *harmful* levels of drinking. In the U.K., 1 unit of alcohol equates to approximately 8 g of alcohol. In the U.S., Canada, Australia, and New Zealand, alcohol is measured in *standard drinks*, equivalent to 10 to 12 g of alcohol. Thus, 3 units of alcohol is approximately equivalent to two standard drinks. From the foregoing, the number of units of alcohol consumed is used to check if patients are in the *safe, increasing risk*, or *harmful* drinking categories.[6] The assumption made here is that *safe limits* for older people are similar to those for younger drinkers. Although professionals may be well aware that these are approximations and are for guidance, the general public tends to adhere to these rather more rigidly. Therefore, the elderly man drinking 21 units of alcohol, despite having problems related to drinking, may not be readily identified as such.

It is estimated that 10 to 15% of those aged 65 and over abuse or are dependent on alcohol.[7] Although the rates of abuse tend to decrease in old age, there are suggestions that projected population changes will result in an increased proportion. In the U.K. in 1994, 15.7% of the population was aged over 65 years whereas that proportion will rise to 25.6% by 2061. This pattern it is estimated will be repeated in most of the Western world and also Japan.[8] As the current adults are aging in an alcohol-tolerant culture, the upcoming cohorts of elderly people are likely to continue to use alcohol. Just how the population dynamics will affect the prevalence of alcohol-related problems in this setting is uncertain.[9] The likelihood, however, is that alcohol-related problems in the elderly population are here to stay and possibly in a big way and may get even bigger.[20]

Different methods of reporting yield different results on the prevalence of this problem. However, general agreement is available in the following areas:

1. Alcohol-related problems among elderly people pose a significant challenge.[10]
2. More men than women are affected.[10]
3. The problem is more prevalent in younger elderly than the older elderly people (60 to 75 years vs. 76 and over).[10]
4. The problem appears to be more prevalent in the hospital population than in the community.
5. Recognition of alcohol-related problems in the elderly population is *poorer* than in younger people.[11,12]
6. Far *fewer* elderly people with alcohol-related problems are referred further for rehabilitation.[2,3,11]

In both young and elderly drinkers, alcohol-related problems may present as *psychological* or *psychiatric, physical,* and *socioeconomic.* In clinical situations, socioeconomic presentations are probably the least common manifestation of alcohol abuse in the elderly population and will not be discussed further.

Psychological/Psychiatric Problems

1. Behavioral changes such as irritability, interpersonal disharmony, and aggression may be why the patient comes to the attention of health-care workers.
2. Psychiatric disorders such as anxiety states, depression, psychotic syndromes such as alcoholic hallucinations or paranoid states or morbid jealousy may be the main manifestation. In addition, self-neglect, as in the senile squalor syndrome, and confusional states, as well as dependency or withdrawal syndromes, can all occur. Although causation is not the issue here, it is worth mentioning the relationship between alcohol abuse and depression. Depressive symptoms in elderly community-based people are common, ranging from 10 to 15%; of whom 1 to 3% also fulfill criteria for major depressive disorder.[13] In addition, the 1992 U.S. household survey showed that among those aged 65 and over who fulfilled DSM-IV criteria for major depression, 13% also met criteria for lifetime alcohol use disorder compared with just 4.5% in nondepressed subjects.[14] Clearly, awareness of the association between depression and alcohol abuse is important. There is currently no firm evidence that alcohol abuse or alcohol dependence causes depressive illness. What is accepted, however, is that even in elderly people, alcohol can worsen depressive illness and also that current drinking is associated with depressive symptoms, which tend to improve on cessation of drinking alcohol. Atkinson[15] has reviewed this issue

more fully, but for the present purposes an important message is that attending health-care workers should be alerted to the possibility of alcohol abuse or dependence in elderly people with depressive symptoms or illness, both of which are common. Acute withdrawal syndromes such as delirium tremens present with both psychiatric and physical correlates. These, together with the cognitive impairments such as Korsakoff syndrome and the acute syndrome of Wernicke's encephalopathy, present in much the same way as they do in younger drinkers. As with younger patients Wernicke's syndrome is reversible if treated early but although some improvement may be had with treatment of Korsakoff syndrome, this is only of the order of 20% of cases.[16] The challenge in the elderly population is therefore to quickly recognize Wernicke's syndrome from among the many possible pathologies that may confound the presentation and Korsakoff syndrome from other causes of memory problems, which are already common in this group.

Physical Problems

Physical problems such as falls, collapses, accidents, gastrointestinal symptoms, fits, or liver/heart failure are often evident. However, the changes of old age modify these complications. Consider this: To develop the alcohol dependence syndrome, a number of conditions need to be met. Among them are that the individual must be robust enough physically for prolonged heavy alcohol intake, and also must have fair or foul means of financing the habit. Few elderly people have sufficient such resources. Their physical and/or financial resources tend to collapse long before frank alcohol dependence develops. It is perhaps no accident that among the elderly population, it is those in the higher socioeconomic stratum who are more likely to develop alcohol dependence.[17] Unlike younger people, elderly people are less likely to fund their drinking through crime or borrowing. The suggestion from the above argument, therefore, is that elderly people who abuse alcohol are more likely to present with physical problems related to their drinking. Research evidence exists to suggest that this may be the case and that this presentation pattern differs from that observed in younger drinkers. Mulinga[2] compared the admission destination between under-60 and over-59 drinkers with ICD-9 alcohol abuse or dependence to a University Hospital over a 4-year period (1992 to 1996). Of the 2524 admission episodes representing 1441 patients under 60, 1968 episodes (78%), representing 912 patients, were admitted to psychiatric services including alcohol therapy units. In contrast, the figures for the over-59 group were 71% to medical or surgical wards and 29% to psychiatric services. Table 5.1 outlines the index diagnoses at admission. The most common presentations were falls (34%) and falls with head injury (28%). Nearly 70% of the presentations were due to some kind of fall

(fall, head injury, collapse, and "off legs"). This finding is in keeping with the expectation that elderly people developing alcohol-related problems would mainly present with physical problems, suggested earlier in the chapter. Many reasons have been given for the low-pickup rate of these problems, including old age changes, multiple pathologies, polypharmacy especially involving psychotropic drugs, as well as poor memory of drinking or of problems, and also relatives' and health-care workers' attitudes.[21] However, ultimately a complete workup including a comprehensive history, examination, and investigation can only be done if the diagnosis is suspected in the first place. It is perhaps unrealistic to expect alcohol histories to be obtained from every elderly patient. Studies such as the above help to focus on where to concentrate our efforts and also to suggest presentations that should raise our index of suspicion about alcohol abuse in the elderly population.

TABLE 5.1

Diagnoses

Initial Presentation	Frequency	Percent	Valid %	Cum. %
Fall	34	27.2	27.2	27.2
Head injury	28	22.4	22.4	49.6
Collapse	13	10.4	10.4	60.0
Ischemic heart disease	10	8.0	8.0	68.0
GI bleed	12	9.6	9.6	77.6
Liver failure	4	3.2	3.2	80.8
Fit	5	4.0	4.0	84.8
Withdrawal	1	0.8	0.8	85.6
RTA	2	1.6	1.6	87.2
Off legs	11	8.8	8.8	85.6
Confusion	5	4.0	4.0	100.0
Total	125	100.0	100.0	
Valid cases	125			
Missing cases	0			

GI = Gastrointestinal; RTA = Road Traffic Accident
Courtesy of John Wiley & Sons Ltd. 1999.

Rehabilitation

Following diagnosis and providing the patient acknowledges the problem and agrees to have intervention, detoxification (where appropriate) and the process of rehabilitation start. Some patients only require and benefit from advice from their doctors (brief intervention).[12] In the U.K., detoxification usually involves the use of the benzodiazepine chlordiazepoxide in a dose range of up to 60 to 100 mg in 24 h, with elderly people recommended half this, together with thiamine orally or parenterally as Pabrinex and vitamin B compound tablets. Because of the risk of anaphylaxis, Pabrinex should only be given where absolutely essential. It should be given over 10 min if given intravenously and should only be administered where facilities for treating anaphylaxis are available.[18] Initial management may also include treatment of other conditions such as anxiety and depression or malnutrition or sorting out a patient's adverse social situation, for example, accommodations. Education about alcohol and its role in alcohol-related problems and group therapy about the cycle of change or relapse prevention are a significant part of rehabilitation. Unfortunately, most facilities for alcohol rehabilitation are designed for younger people. Elderly patients are disadvantaged in feeling out of place, may not quite keep pace with the rest of the group, and some of the discussions may not be relevant to their situation, and vice versa. The way forward seems to be the creation of age-specific facilities for elderly patients. Evidence exists to suggest that indeed the elderly patient with alcohol-related problems would do better in such a facility.[7,19] However, our enthusiasm for this should be tempered by our currently poor ability to identify alcohol problems in this age group in the first instance, and also by the seeming inertia in referring diagnosed patients on for rehabilitation.[2,3]

Several drug preparations are available to help maintain abstinence. Disulfiram (Antabuse), an acetaldehyde dehydrogenase inhibitor, helps maintain abstinence by causing unpleasant symptoms when alcohol is concurrently consumed through the accumulation of acetaldehyde. Unfortunately, the adverse drug reactions associated with disulfiram make it a less useful drug in the elderly patient. For instance, it is contraindicated in those with coronary artery and cerebrovascular disease, which are common in elderly people. Acamprosate calcium and naltrexone are anticraving drugs for alcohol. Naltrexone is not available for this purpose in the U.K. Although acamprosate calcium is available for use, it is currently only licensed for those aged 18 to 65.[18] For those requiring more prolonged rehabilitation, "dry" or half-way houses may be beneficial. Others may require only counseling from their doctors, nurses, or psychologists. Attendance at Alcoholics Anonymous (AA) meetings may also be helpful. It is, however, useful to remember that elderly patients may be better managed in their own homes with support in familiar surroundings and family or friends if possible. But this approach may be inappropriate for patients living alone or those requiring hospital intervention or those with a history of withdrawal fits.

Case History

A 77-year-old married woman presented to the emergency room having fallen down a staircase. The fall had occurred in the morning as she tried to get downstairs. She was observed for 12 h and then discharged home. A week later her personal doctor was called to see her because she had collapsed. There was a strong smell of alcohol, but no other findings were reported. A few days later a referral to an old age psychiatrist was made, because the woman had become agitated, aggressive, and had threatened to hit her husband of 56 years with a hammer.

It became apparent she had been drinking at least two bottles of brandy per week, and her husband bought these for her to keep the peace. She had had numerous falls and blackouts previously. Although this had gone on for years and she had gone to the accident and emergency department on many occasions, the diagnosis had remained "elusive" and she had never had any intervention. On this occasion, she readily acknowledged her problem and entered a community rehabilitation program. In her case, this involved education of both the patient and her husband of the link between her level of drinking and her falls and blackouts as well as the aggressive outbursts. She was also given a supervised chlordiazepoxide regime and multivitamins. This was then followed by a referral to her local Community Alcohol Team for further support and relapse prevention.

This case highlights the difficulties in the care of elderly people with alcohol problems:

1. Difficulties in picking up the problem
2. Difficulties family members may have in accepting and reporting such a problem
3. Delays in appropriate referrals

This woman was referred not because of her alcohol problem but because she threatened her husband with a hammer. The referring agent had requested that she be considered for formal admission under a section of the Mental Health Act. However, alcohol intoxication/withdrawal in the absence of mental illness is not covered under the Mental Health Act.

Conclusion

A lot of evidence suggests that alcohol-related problems are common but are poorly recognized in elderly people. Sadly, even when identified, such patients do not seem to be referred on for rehabilitation despite evidence that they benefit from such intervention. Elderly people, because of age-associated changes, may present differently with alcohol-related problems. The current approach to diagnosis, treatment, and rehabilitation relies to a great extent on information obtained in younger people (18 to 64 years), which may not necessarily be the best for elderly people. The challenges that healthcare workers for the elderly population face include improved recognition of alcohol-related problems in this group and also referral for appropriate rehabilitation. The key to meeting these challenges is the conduct of age-specific research; such research would improve recognition of alcohol-related problems in elderly people, establish such issues as "safe" drinking levels, and also allow the elderly to benefit from safe pharmaceutical preparations just as younger drinkers do from disulfiram, acamprosate calcium, or naltrexone.

Acknowledgments

The author is grateful for the help in typing by Miss J. Pickup.

References

1. Lucey, M.R., Hill, E.M., Young, J.P. et al., The influences of age and gender on blood ethanol concentration in healthy humans, *J. Stud. Alcohol.*, 60, 103–110, 1999.
2. Mulinga, J., Elderly people with alcohol-related problems: where do they go? *Int. J. Geriatr. Psychiatr.*, 14, 564–566, 1999.
3. McInnes, E. and Powell, J., Drug and alcohol referrals: are elderly substance diagnoses and referrals being missed? *Br. Med. J.*, 308, 444–446.
4. Gronbaek, M., Deis, A., Becker, U. et al., Alcohol and mortality: is there a U-shaped relation in elderly people? *Age Aging*, 27, 739–744.
5. Lindeman, R.D., Romero, L.J. Allen, A.S. et al., Alcohol consumption is negatively associated with the prevalence of coronary heart disease in the New Mexico elder health survey, *J. Am. Geriatr. Soc.*, 47, 396–401, 1999.
6. Royal College of Physicians, Psychiatrists and General Practitioners, Alcohol and the Heart in Perspective: Sensible Limits Reaffirmed, Report of a Joint Working Group, 1995.
7. Zimberg, S., Treating alcoholism: an age specific intervention that works for older patients, *Geriatrics*, 51, 45–49, 1996.
8. House of Commons Health Committee, Long Term Care: Future Provision and Funding, 1, 26–28, 1996.
9. Nirenberg, T.D., Lisansky-Gomberg, E.S., and Cellucci, T., Substance abuse disorders, in *Handbook of Clinical Geropsychology*, Hersen, M. and VanHasselt, V.B., Eds., Plenum Press, New York, 1998, 147–172.
10. Atkinson, R.M., Alcoholism and drug abuse in the elderly, in Jacoby, R. and Oppenheimer, C., Eds., Oxford Medical Publications, Oxford, 1996, Chap. 23.
11. Thibault, J.M. and Maly, R.C., Recognition and treatment of substance abuse in the elderly, *Substance Abuse*, 20, 155–165, 1993.
12. Ashworth, M. and Gerada, C., Addiction and dependency/alcohol, in *ABC of Mental Health*, Davies, T. and Craig, T.K.J., Eds., BMJ Books, London, 2000, Chap. 12.
13. Baldwin, R.C., Depressive illness in psychiatry in the elderly, in Jacoby, R. and Oppenheimer, C., Eds., Oxford Medical Publications, Oxford, 1996, Chap. 19.

14. Grant, B.F. and Harford, T.C., Comorbidity between DSM-IV alcohol use disorders and major depression: results of a national survey, *Drug Alcohol Dependence*, 39, 197–206, 1995.
15. Atkinson, R.M., Depression, alcoholism and aging: a review, *Int. J. Geriatr. Psychiatr.*, 14, 905–910, 1999.
16. Kaplan, H.I. and Sadock, B.J., Alcohol-related disorders, in *Synopsis of Psychiatry*, Kaplan H.I. and Sadock, B.J., Eds., 1999, Chap. 12.
17. Cohen, G., Fleming, N.F., Glatter, K.A. et al., Epidemiology of substance misuse, in *Source Book of Substance Misuse and Addiction*, Friedman, L., Fleming, N.F., Roberts, D.H., and Hyman, S.E., Eds., Williams and Wilkins, Baltimore, 1996, Chap. 2.
18. *British National Formulary*, 38, Sept. 1999.
19. Kofoed, L.L., Tolson, R.L., Atkinson, R.M. et al., Treatment compliance of older alcoholics: an elder specific approach is superior to "mainstreaming," *J. Stud. Alcohol.*, 48, 47, 1987.
20. Moore, A.A., Hays, R.D., Greendale, G.A., Damesyn, M., and Reuben, D.B., Drinking habits among older persons, findings from NHANES 1 epidemiologic follow up study (1982–1984), *J. Am. Geriatri. Soc.*, 47, 412–416, 1999.
21. Egbert, A.M., The older alcoholic: recognising the subtle clinical clues, *Geriatrics*, 48, 63–67, 1993.

6

Coffee, Tea, and Hypertension in Elderly People

Robert Eggertsen and Åke Andreasson

CONTENTS

Introduction

Coffee has been one of the most-used stimulants for many years. One of the compounds in coffee is caffeine, which chemically is a methylxanthine, and is partly responsible for the cardiovascular influence of coffee on heart rate and blood pressure. Caffeine, administered acutely after abstinence, increases blood pressure, catecholamines, and plasma renin activity in normotensive individuals.[1,2] During habitual ingestion, tolerance to the hemodynamic and humoral effects of caffeine seems to develop in normotensive subjects.[3] The influence of caffeine on blood pressure was investigated for the first time in 1934, when experiments were conducted on young volunteers.[4] Since then, several trials have been conducted, but, as a number of them were not performed as controlled studies, safe conclusions are difficult to draw. The different ways of preparing coffee, such as brewing and boiling, have also complicated interpretation of the health effects. Population studies have shown increased s-cholesterol in people using boiled coffee, which together with pressor effects theoretically could enhance the cardiovascular influence. There is also caffeine in tea but to a much smaller extent; in a regular cup of tea the content of caffeine is about 40

0-8493-2257-X/01/$0.00+$.50
© 2001 by CRC Press LLC

mg compared with 100 to 150 mg caffeine in a cup of coffee.[6] As with several hypertension studies, few studies have focused on an elderly population. The same circumstances are valid for trials of the hypertensive effects of coffee and tea, and this chapter discusses caffeine effects of coffee and tea in elderly people, those both with and without hypertension.

Effects on Normotensive Individuals

In a meta-analysis in 1999 of 36 studies on chronic coffee drinking and blood pressure, only 11 trials met sufficient criteria, with control groups and relevant study design.[5] The results indicated that there was a small effect with an increase of 2.4 mmHg on systolic blood pressure and 1.2 mmHg on diastolic blood pressure during chronic coffee consumption, but that this effect was more pronounced in younger people. Because the investigations only had a duration of 14 to 79 days, longer trials, combined with other risk factors, should be performed to confirm the results. This is important because after a short time an adaptation to the pressor effects occurs,[3] which indicates that longer duration trials are needed to decide if these effects influence cardiovascular morbidity. Very few elderly people were recruited for the 11 studies, and 10 studies were done on individuals without antihypertensive medication. In another trial on elderly normotensive people with a mean age of 72.1 years (range 54 to 89 years), 22 normotensive people were compared with 26 hypertensive individuals. Blood pressure was measured with ambulatory blood pressure monitoring (ABPM), and in the normotensive group no significant effects on blood pressure or heart rate were established when comparison was made between a caffeine-free diet and coffee.[7] Problems with postural and postprandial hypotension in elderly people can predispose them to falls. In a study of 171 subjects with a mean age of 75.2 years (range 53 to 95 years), the postprandial fall of blood pressure in the normotensive coffee-drinking group (n = 62) showed an attenuation of the significant reduction in supine and standing blood pressure.[8]

Similar effects were demonstrated in earlier trials on elderly people,[9,10] indicating habitual coffee drinking could be a valuable tool against intermittent falls of blood pressure. The caffeine effects of tea drinking are contradictory, with both decreasing and unchanged blood pressure.[11,12] There could also be differences between black and green tea because of their different polyphenolic compositions.[13] Only rat studies have been performed thus far with green tea extracts, and those results suggest a lowering of blood pressure.[14] No studies have focused solely on elderly normotensive people. One trial, with a mean age of 56 years (range 35 to 73 years), that measured the acute effects showed a short rise in blood pressure at 30 min, but changes after 60 min and during ABPM were not significant. This study also showed no significant differences between black and green tea.[15]

Effects on Hypertensive Patients

The above-mentioned meta-analysis[5] comprised 11 trials, but only one with hypertensive subjects. In this study, 23 men and women with a mean age of 56 years (range 28 to 74) participated and blood pressure measurements were made with ABPM.[16] There appeared to be no evidence that habitual coffee intake influenced blood pressure in treated patients with hypertension.[16] This was in contrast to the other trials on normotensive people in the meta-analysis, which showed a slight increase in the coffee-drinking group.[5] In a small study with eight patients with hypertension with a mean age of 75 years (range 65 to 82), the acute effects of caffeine were determined and showed a small increase in blood pressure after 48 h of caffeine abstention, which was not seen after a shorter period of 12 h.[17] In a study with 63 treated hypertensive subjects with a mean age of 77 years, the postprandial fall of supine and standing blood pressure was not significantly changed.[8] This was in contrast to a group of 46 untreated hypertensive people with a mean age of 76.6 years where abstainers of coffee showed a significant attenuation of postprandial supine systolic blood pressure.[8] In the same trial, tea drinkers with treated hypertension also experienced an attenuation of the supine and standing systolic blood pressure.[8] If caffeine is administered 60 min or more before a meal, the postprandial fall in blood pressure is not prevented in elderly people.[18] If any effect is to be achieved, it seems the caffeine must be ingested 30 min before or immediately after the meal.[9,10] Postprandial hypotension in elderly people occurs at a maximum of 60 min after eating. The decrease in blood pressure reaches its maximum effect after 30 to 60 min,[19] at which time peak plasma levels are achieved.[20]

Effects on Cardiovascular Morbidity and Mortality

Coffee has been implicated as a potential risk factor for cardiovascular disease, but the results from different population studies are contradictory.[21-23] Studies focusing only on an elderly population are not usual, but one cross-sectional Australian study with 843 subjects aged 60 to 87 years found an independent association between coffee drinking and diastolic blood pressure in men and women with treated hypertension.[24] In a Dutch population comprising 255 individuals aged 65 to 79 years a positive correlation existed between coffee consumption and systolic and diastolic blood pressure in women, but this could partly depend on increased urinary excretion of calcium, sodium, and potassium.[25,26] Hypertensive men in the Honolulu Heart Program in older middle age (55 to 68 years) appeared to have an increased risk of developing thromboembolic stroke when drinking three or more cups of coffee per day compared with nondrinkers.[27] The results should be confirmed in other trials because of the small number of stroke events. A weak association between cardiovascular disease and mortality was seen in a study of males belonging to the Seventh-Day Adventists, but the association decreased with age.[28] The men were followed up from age 50 to 53 years to age 73 to 78 years and up to 10% were hypertensive. The results were supported by a Norwegian study,[29] but in a Swedish cohort of middle-aged men no such relation was demonstrated.[22] Nor did the Hypertension Detection and Follow-up Program with 10,000 subjects with hypertension aged 30 to 69 years provide evidence that coffee consumption is related to increased mortality rates.[30] Investigations with decaffeinated coffee in Italian women aged 24 to 69 years with acute myocardial infarction showed no benefit compared with regular coffee consumption in reducing infarction risk.[31]

Conclusions

Caffeine, in coffee and tea, has been used worldwide for hundreds of years as a weak stimulant. Several studies have focused on its influence on blood pressure, and effects have been demonstrated with an increased pressure of small magnitude. The results are, however, not unequivocal, and most studies have been performed on younger age groups. The effects of caffeine on cardiovascular morbidity and mortality have therefore been studied in different cohorts of older people around the world, and here also the results are contradictory. Caffeine could also have positive consequences on blood pressure in an elderly population, because a postprandial fall of pressure could be attenuated by caffeine. Against this background stand the social aspects of coffee and tea consumption, a benefit that, in the elderly population will probably outweigh any eventual small negative influences of caffeine on blood pressure.

References

1. Robertson, D., Fröhlich, J., Carr, K., Watson, J., Hollifield, J., Shand, D., and Oates, J., Effects of caffeine on plasma renin activity, catecholamines and blood pressure, *N. Engl. J. Med.*, 298, 181, 1978.
2. Casiglia, E., Bongiovi, S., Paleari, C.D., Petucco, S., Boni, M., Colangeli, G., Penzo, M., and Pessina, A.C., Haemodynamic effects of coffee and caffeine in normal volunteers: a placebo-controlled clinical study, *J. Int. Med.*, 229, 501, 1991.

3. Robertson, D., Wase, D., Workman, R., Woosley, R., and Oates, J., Tolerance to the humoral and haemodynamic effects of caffeine in man, *J. Clin. Invest.*, 67, 1111, 1981.
4. Horst, K., Buxton, R.E., and Robinson, W.D., The effect of the habitual use of coffee or decaffeinated coffee upon blood pressure and certain motor reactions of normal young men, *J. Pharmacol. Exp. Ther.*, 52, 322, 1934.
5. Jee, S.H., Hee, J., Whelton, P.K., Suh, I., and Klag, M.J., The effect of chronic coffee drinking on blood pressure. A meta-analysis of controlled clinical trials, *Hypertension*, 33, 647, 1999.
6. Scott, N.R., Chakraborty, J., and Marks, V., Caffeine consumption in the United Kingdom: a retrospective survey, *Food Sci. Nutr.*, 42F, 183, 1989.
7. Rakic, V., Burke, V., and Beilin, L.J., Effects of coffee on ambulatory pressure in older men and women. A randomized controlled trial, *Hypertension*, 33, 869, 1999.
8. Rakic, V., Beilin, L.J., and Burke, V., Effect of coffee and tea drinking on postprandial hypotension in older men and women, *Clin. Exp. Pharmacol. Physiol.*, 23, 559, 1996.
9. Heseltine, D., Dakkak, M., Woodhouse, K., Macdonald, I.A., and Potter, J.F., The effect of caffeine on postprandial hypotension in the elderly, *J. Am. Geriatr. Soc.*, 39, 160, 1991.
10. Heseltine, D., El-Jabri, M., Ahmed, K., and Knox, J., The effect of caffeine on postprandial blood pressure in the frail elderly, *Postgrad. Med. J.*, 67, 543, 1991.
11. Stenswold, I., Terdal, A., Solvol, K., and Foss, O.P., Tea consumption. Relationship to cholesterol, blood pressure and coronary and total mortality, *Prev. Med.*, 21, 546, 1992.
12. Bingham, S.A., Vorster, H., Jerling, J.C., Magee, E., Mulligan, A., Runswick, S.A. et al., Effect of tea drinking on blood lipids, blood pressure and aspects of bowel habit, *Br. J. Nutr.*, 78, 41, 1997.
13. Ballantine, D.A., Wiseman, S.A., and Bouwens, L.C.M., The chemistry of tea flavonoids, *Crit. Rev. Food Sci. Nutr.*, 37, 693, 1997.
14. Abe, Y., Umemura, S., Sugomoto, K., Hirawa, N., Kato, Y., Yokohama, N. et al., Effect of green tea rich in gamma-aminobutyric acid on blood pressure of Dahl-sensitive rats, *Am. J. Hypertens.*, 8, 74, 1995.
15. Hodgson, J., Puddey, I., Burke, V., Beilin, L., and Jordan, N., Effects on blood pressure of drinking green and black tea, *J. Hypertension*, 17, 457, 1999.
16. Eggertsen, R., Andreasson, Å., Hedner, T., Karlberg, B.E., and Hansson, L., Effect of coffee on ambulatory blood pressure in patients with treated hypertension, *J. Int. Med.*, 233, 351, 1993.
17. Potter, J.F., Haigh, R.A., Harper, G.D., Fotherby, M., Hurd, S., and Macdonald, I.A., Blood pressure, plasma catecholamine and renin responses to caffeine in elderly hypertensives, *J. Hum. Hypertens.*, 7, 273, 1993.
18. Lenders, J.W.M., Morre, H.L.C., Smits, P., and Thien, T., The effects of caffeine on the postprandial fall of blood pressure in the elderly, *Age Ageing*, 17, 236, 1988.
19. Onrot, J., Goldberg, M. R., Biaggione, I., Hollister, A. S., Kincaid, D., and Robertson, D., Hemodynamic and humoral effects of caffeine in autonomic failure, *N. Engl. J. Med.*, 313, 549, 1985.
20. Smits, P., Thien, Th., and van't Laar, A., Circulatory effects of coffee in relation to the pharmacokinetics of caffeine, *Am. J. Cardiol.*, 56, 958, 1985.

21. Grobbee, D., Rimm, E., Giovannucci, E., Colditz, G., Stampfer, M., and Willet, W., Coffee, caffeine, and cardiovascular disease in men, *N. Engl. J. Med.*, 323, 1026, 1990.

22. Rosengren, A. and Wilhelmsen, L., Coffee, coronary heart disease and mortality in middle-aged Swedish men: finding from the Primary Prevention Study, *J. Int. Med.*, 230, 67, 1991.

23. Wilson, P.W.F., Garrison, R., Kannel, W.B., McGee, D.L., and Catelli, W.P., Is coffee consumption a contributor to cardiovascular disease? Insights from the Framingham Study, *Arch. Intern. Med.*, 149, 1169, 1989.

24. Burke, V., Beilin, R., German, R., Grosskopf, S., Ritchie, J., Puddey, I.B., and Rogers, P., Association of lifestyle and personality characteristics with blood pressure and hypertension: a cross-sectional study in the elderly, *J. Clin. Epidemiol.*, 45, 1061, 1992.

25. Löwik, M., Hofman, Z., Kok, F., Wedel, M., Hulshof, K., Odink, J., and Schaafsmaa, G., Nutrition and blood pressure among elderly men and women (Dutch Nutrition Surveillance System), *J. Am. Coll. Nutr.*, 10, 149, 1991.

26. Massey, L.K. and Wise, K.J., The effect of dietary caffeine on urinary excretion of calcium, magnesium, sodium and potassium in healthy young females, *Nutr. Res.*, 4, 43, 1984.

27. Hakim, A.A., Ross, G.W., Curb, J.D., Rodriguez, B.L., Burchfiel, C.M., Sharp, D.S., Yano, K., and Abbott, R.D., Coffee consumption in hypertensive men in older middle-age and the risk of stroke: the Honolulu Heart Program, *J. Clin. Epidemiol.*, 51, 487, 1998.

28. Lindsted, K.D., Kuzma, J.W., and Anderson, J.L., Coffee consumption and cause-specific mortality. Association with age and death and compression of mortality, *J. Clin. Epidemiol.*, 45, 733, 1992.

29. Tverdal, A., Stensvold, I., Solvoll, K., Foss, O., Lund-Larsen, P., and Bjartveit, K., Coffee consumption and death from coronary heart disease in middle-aged Norwegian men and women, *Br. Med. J.*, 300, 566, 1990.

30. Martin, J.B., Annegers, F.J., Curb, D.J., Heyden, S., Howson, C., Lee, E.S., and Lee, M., Mortality patterns among hypertensives by reported level of caffeine consumption, *Prev. Med.*, 17, 310, 1988.

31. La Vecchia, C., Dávanzo, B., Negri, E., Franceschi, S., Gentile, A., and Tavani, A., Decaffeinated coffee and acute myocardial infarction. A case-control study in Italian women, *Ann. Epidemiol.*, 3, 601, 1993.

7

Caffeine and Insomnia in Elderly People

Hilary A. Wynne

CONTENTS

Caffeine

Caffeine is the world's most ubiquitously used drug, with 96% of an American population having ever used and 83% at present using, one or more caffeinated beverages weekly.[1] Every year, an estimated 120,000 tonnes of caffeine are consumed globally. Most of this is derived from tea and coffee (54 and 43%, respectively), with chocolate and soft drinks making other significant contributions. Pharmaceutical preparations account for less than 1% of global consumption. Intake shows intraindividual variation, with habitual intake in a postmenopausal female U.S. population estimated to range from 0 to 1400 mg/day.[2] Prospective food records can overestimate caffeine intake compared with chemical analysis of brewed beverage, however. Tobacco, caffeine, and alcohol use tends to co-occur in adults, including older men and women.[3]

Current intake is a poor measurement of lifetime intake. Of ever-users of caffeine in Vermont, 41% had stopped at least one type of caffeinated beverage, and 14% had stopped caffeine altogether, mostly due to health concerns

0-8493-2257-X/01/$0.00+$.50
© 2001 by CRC Press LLC

and unpleasant side effects.[1] A study of a U.S. population, mean age 64 years (range 30 to 105 years), that had reduced caffeinated coffee intake, showed respondents had begun drinking caffeinated coffee around age 20 and decaffeinated coffee around age 50. More women than men had decided to curtail caffeinated coffee, and more women did so because of sleep problems, while more men did so because their spouses stopped drinking it. Most people had done so on their own initiative, 80% for health concerns, with only 10% doing so on advice from a physician.[4]

Pharmacokinetics

Caffeine is a methylxanthine, which, along with other xanthines, theobromine and theophylline, is widely distributed in food. After ingestion, it is rapidly and almost totally absorbed from the gastrointestinal tract, with a peak concentration of around 30 to 60 min depending on the presence or absence of food. Because of the greater proportion of adipose tissue to lean body mass, a dose of caffeine expressed as milligram per kilogram total body weight is likely to result in higher plasma and tissue concentrations in elderly people compared with younger individuals. The major route of metabolism is by hepatic N-demethylation to methylxanthines, followed by acetylation. In humans, the half-life of elimination ($t_{1/2}$) averages between 4 and 6 h, but there is a wide interindividual variation, with ranges from 2 to 12 h in healthy adults being common.[5] There is evidence that caffeine metabolism is dose dependent, and it accumulates with chronic and frequent ingestion.[6] Schnegg and Lauterburg[7] found caffeine clearance to be lower by 35% in 13 healthy elderly subjects in comparison with young subjects. Cigarette smoking accelerates caffeine metabolism by around 50%,[8] whereas the oral contraceptive pill produces an average of a 33% fall, although there is no gender effect upon metabolism.

Pharmacodynamics

The effects of caffeine are mediated by a reversible blockade of adenosine receptors. Adenosine is an intermediary of a wide range of metabolic pathways. It has effects on two main classes of receptors, an A1 (high-affinity) receptor and an A2 (low-affinity) receptor. Activation of the A1 results in inhibition of adenylate cyclase, whereas an excitatory effect is thought to be mediated by the A2 receptor.[9] Caffeine antagonizes both receptors at physiological concentrations. As the affinity for the A1 is greater than for the A2 receptor, the overall effect of antagonism is to overcome inhibition of adenylate cyclase activity, leading to increased concentrations of cyclic AMP and central stimulation via neurotransmitter release.

Many approaches and measures have been used to assess the effects of caffeine on performance and sleep. Some of the literature about the physiological and behavioral effects of caffeine is difficult to interpret, probably because studies are confounded by a number of factors. As caffeine is almost universally taken by adults in varying doses, who possibly have acquired pharmacokinetic and pharmacodynamic tolerance; this, superimposed on variability in experimental design, could affect the outcome of studies. Perceived actions could be the result of the direct effects of caffeine, or its indirect effects through removal of withdrawal symptoms after a period of caffeine deprivation (often overnight), all affected by time of study and the personalities of the subjects studied. Although it is generally accepted that caffeine quickens reaction time, enhances vigilance performance, increases self-perceived alertness, and improves mood, the direct beneficial effects of caffeine, or resolving caffeine deprivation, may both contribute. Results can also be inconsistent, as studies may not have been capable of measuring the complex effects of the drug on individual performance. Designs may fail to take into account the general rule that complicated tasks are performed better at low levels of arousal, and simple tasks at higher levels of arousal.

To summarize caffeine stimulatory action, caffeine helps to maintain speed and accuracy at lower doses, but may impair fine-motor control at higher doses; it increases alertness, vigilance, concentration, and agitation self-ratings; and it reduces fatigue and relaxation self-rating relative to a placebo.[10] Recently, the term *caffeinism* has been introduced and used in connection with a syndrome that closely resembles the clinical manifestations of anxiety, with insomnia, nervousness, irritability, tremulousness, tachycardia, and gastrointestinal symptoms, and has been shown to be associated with high caffeine use.[11] Caffeine is capable of producing a mild degree of addiction, and it is possible to demonstrate discrimination between caffeine and placebo in humans.[12] In addition, upon withdrawal, a characteristic abstinence syndrome, which may resemble anxiety (headache, increased nervousness, lethargy, and restlessness), has been demonstrated.[11] These symptoms rapidly disappear on the resumption of caffeine intake.

Age-Related Pharmacodynamic Changes

Age-associated pharmacodynamic changes occur, with evidence suggesting that elderly people are more sensitive to the objectively measured effects upon performance, but report fewer subjectively felt effects. While young people felt more alert, calmer, more interested, and steadier on caffeine, no such effect was reported by the elderly.[13] In a study of the relationship of blood pressure, heart rate, behavior, and mood state to norepinephrine kinetics in young (19 to 26 years) and elderly (65 to 80 years) healthy men following ingestion of 5 mg/kg fat-free mass of caffeine, systolic and diastolic blood pressure increased significantly by 9 and 3% in older men following caffeine ingestion, but remained unchanged in younger men. Self-reported feelings of tension and anger decreased in older men, while anger tended to increase in younger men, suggesting that elderly people are more reactive to the pressor and less sensitive to the subjective effects of caffeine. These were not mediated by changes in norepinephrine kinetics.[14] In a study of the dose–response relationship upon psychomotor performance of caffeine and theophylline in healthy elderly volunteers, a significant improvement on a continuous attention task was seen at the lowest concentration of caffeine and theophylline used, while at higher concentrations there was a nonsignificant trend toward placebo scores. Caffeine had a lack of effect upon subjective measures, as in previous studies.[15] The suggestion that caffeine may enhance cognitive performance to a greater extent in older than in young adults has not been universally supported.[16]

Sleep

Sleeping and waking feeling refreshed eludes many of us. Given the wide variation in sleep habits, insomnia has been given a subjective definition as "a feeling by an individual that he or she is not obtaining sufficient, or good quality sleep, despite ample opportunity to sleep." Sleep quality can be assessed subjectively using sleep questionnaires such as the Pittsburgh Sleep Quality Index.[17]

Although our understanding of arousal and sleep-promoting systems is incomplete, insomnia can be associated with factors that either increase activity in the arousal systems of the brain, including the ascending reticular activating or limbic arousal systems, or decrease activity in the sleep-promoting areas, including those located in the pons. The sleep architecture is very sensitive to both exogenous (e.g., noise, caffeine) and endogenous factors (e.g., depression). The incidence of chronic insomnia is high, and rises with age, with between 10 and 45% of people surveyed reporting insomnia.[18] This is the result of both changes intrinsic to aging and external environmental influences.

Age-Related Changes in Sleep Pattern

The requirement for sleep varies. Most people, undisturbed, would sleep for 7 to 9 h/24-h period. The sleep of the older person is disturbed more than in youth, with a reduction in the amount of nonrapid eye movement (non REM) sleep, especially in the deepest (EEG slow wave) sleep.[19] Elderly people also spend spend more time awake in bed,[20] and the subjective feeling of a longer time waiting for sleep is confirmed by laboratory measurements of a greater sleep latency and more arousals during the night in older adults.

Bixler et al.[21] estimated that 23% of 18 to 30 year olds and 38% of 51 to 80 year olds had a self-perceived problem falling asleep, staying asleep, or awakening too early. Women are more likely to report a subjective sleep problem, with women approximately twice as likely as men to be prescribed sleeping medication.

Caffeine and Insomnia

Caffeine increases the time it takes to fall asleep and the time it takes to obtain deep sleep. Total sleep time is reduced, and there is a relative increase in the proportion of light sleep as opposed to rapid eye movement (REM) and deep sleep.[22] Colton et al.[23] reported that users of caffeine seemed less susceptible to its sleep-disturbing properties than nonusers, inferring the development of tolerance to this effect with use. In a study of the effect of moderate intake of caffeine after caffeine ingestion or abstinence, performance was impaired by withdrawal after habitual use, but seemed not to improve performance with acute or habitual use. Acute ingestion made participants feel more alert and less tired, but less alert following chronic exposure, with reports of sleeping longer and more soundly with caffeine withdrawal. Studies attempting to link caffeine usage to poor sleep have used either an epidemiological or an experimental approach, although there has been little work specific in elderly people.

In a large epidemiological study of 4558 Australians, aged 20 to 70, it was found that the proportion of subjects reporting insomnia, indigestion, palpitations, tremor, and headache increased significantly with mean caffeine intake.[24] The association between these symptoms and usual daily caffeine consumption remained significant in both males and females for palpitations, tremor, headache, and insomnia, after controlling for the potential confounding factors of age, adiposity, smoking, alcohol intake, and occupation. Associations between caffeine intake and symptoms did not depend on the source of caffeine. If the associations are causal, the authors estimated that approximately one quarter of the reported prevalence of palpitations, tremor, headache, and insomnia was attributable to caffeine intake in this population. Although the mechanism of action of caffeine is unknown, it has been shown that serotonin and catecholamine levels are raised by caffeine and these and other CNS metabolites are critically involved in the sleep process. This study failed to show any significant association between reports of insomnia and the time caffeine was consumed before bed. This lack of association may be explained by the long half-life of caffeine.

Older people, particularly women, are more prone to report sleep disturbance, especially if they have mental health problems.[25] Severe daytime sleepiness is associated with females, middle age, napping, insomnia symptoms, high daily caffeine intake, breathing pauses or leg pain in sleep, and depressive disorders in the British population.[26] An association between reported tea consumption and persistent complaints of poor sleep has been reported in elderly people in the community, although plasma caffeine levels were not measured.[27]

In an investigation into the somatic manifestations of caffeine in 124 general hospital patients, higher consumers were older. The age-related increase in use is possibly the result of caffeine tolerance developing after years or decades of gradually increased use.[28] Among the subjects, somatic symptoms including insomnia, anxiety, and tremulousness were common, with some dose–response associations being apparent, with tolerance, if it had developed, being overridden by increased intake of caffeine.

One survey of 181 elderly community-based subjects and 53 elderly patients receiving hospital care found a significant negative correlation between age and coffee, but not tea consumption. Sleep quality deteriorates significantly with age. For the 87 community-dwelling population, in whom late afternoon caffeine concentrations were measured, caffeine concentrations were negatively correlated with sleep quality score, such that levels were lower in those with poorer sleep quality. In the hospital population, median caffeine concentration was higher in patients reporting sleep problems than those without.[29] Self-reported consumption of tea or coffee did not correlate with plasma caffeine concentrations. The findings may be the result of insomniacs residing in the community recognizing the adverse effects of caffeine upon sleep, and restricting intake, whereas institutionalized individuals, who have less control over their environment, do not.

In an experimental approach, looking at caffeine pharmacokinetics in six people declaring themselves as "suffering from caffeine-induced wakefulness," the caffeine-sensitive group has a significantly prolonged elimination half-life for caffeine when compared with the control group.[30] No tests for pharmacodynamic response to caffeine were carried out so a possible pharmacodynamic difference in sensitivity to caffeine cannot be excluded. Due to the small number of subjects and the differing patterns of caffeine intake in the two groups, the authors could not distinguish between the possibility that the slow metabolism in poor sleepers was the result of a lack of pharmacokinetic tolerance or of an innate difference in pharmacokinetics, with impaired metabolism leading to an increased likelihood of sleep problems.

Karacans et al.[22] found in 18 normal young adult males, that a one cup equivalent of regular coffee taken half an hour before bedtime had little or no effect on objective or subjective characteristics of sleep, and a dose-dependent relationship between caffeine and sleep disturbance.[22] Caffeine administered 30 min before bedtime in two to four cup equivalents caused dose-related changes in most standard electroencephalogram–electrooculogram sleep parameters, and caused REM sleep to shift to the early part of the night and stage 3 and 4 sleep to shift to the later parts. It also produced dose-related changes in subjective estimates of sleep characteristics.

Drug withdrawal symptoms are an additional adverse effect of caffeine consumption. That symptoms are relieved by resumption of caffeine intake serves to maintain consumption. The effects of caffeine withdrawal on nocturnal enuresis, use of behavior requiring physical or pharmacological restraint, and insomnia were studied in 30 psychiatric patients, 10 selected for each of the problem areas, the ages of whom were not reported.[31] As a result of several weeks withdrawal, there was a significant reduction in the number of restraints used per week, nocturnal enuresis declined, and reductions of awakenings and sleep medication requests occurred for all patients. The authors recommended that caffeine intake should be stopped several hours before bedtime, to reduce the probability of insomnia. The study is small, and a double blind procedure was not used, introducing the possibility of observer bias.

A study of the effect of caffeine-free beverages on sleep profiles of elderly patients receiving continuing care in the hospital revealed that although caffeine levels fell as a result of a change from caffeine-containing to caffeine-free beverages, no change in sleep pattern was noted overall in the 28 patients studied. Of the 12 patients with sleep problems, identified by sleep questionnaire, a benefit in sleep quality was reported by two individuals, one of whom had been prescribed hypnotics from which she subsequently withdrew.[32]

Beginning in middle age, many normal people who do not complain of insomnia exhibit some electronically measured characteristics that are also exhibited by persons who complain of insomnia. As insomnia incidence and prevalence increase with age, the normal age-related change in sleep mechanisms may make older people especially vulnerable to perturbation by internal or external stimuli. This hypothesis that older individuals are more sensitive to the sleep-disturbing effects of caffeine and coffee has been supported by a comparative study.[33]

Restless leg syndrome is also a very common disorder in the elderly. This is a feeling of discomfort in the lower extremities, which the individual then moves to relieve symptoms. Caffeine may be an aggravating cause, and withdrawal may offer a resolution of the problem, which may be causing insomnia indirectly.[34] Periodic limb movement disorder is a common disorder of the elderly, characterized by repetitive extremity movements. Prevalence is estimated to be around 5% of the population, but between 30 and 40% of elderly people.[35] It causes arousal in both the victim and a bed partner. The disorder is aggravated by caffeine and may be relieved by withdrawal. In a United Kingdom-based study of disordered breathing in 5000 men and women aged 15 to 100 years, who formed a representative sample of the non-institutionalized population, regular snoring was associated with factors including being age 25 or more, male, nighttime awakenings, and consuming large amounts of caffeine.[36]

The effect of temazepam on insomnia effected by caffeine has been studied in young male subjects. A reduction in total sleep time and total amount of REM sleep, and an increase in sleep latency and wake time were observed after caffeine intake, and administration of 15 g or 30 mg of temazepam caused almost complete recovery from this sleep disturbance.[37] A similar result was found in a study of the interaction of caffeine with pentobarbital as a night hypnotic, in a study group of 41 men and 1 woman, mean age 46 years, who were medical or surgical hospital inpatients. In this study, the adverse effects of 250 mg of oral caffeine on sleep were negated by 100 mg oral pentobarbital.[38]

Conclusion

Caffeine intake is almost ubiquitous. A consistently adverse effect of caffeine on sleep is reported and withdrawal is suggested. This, together with the age-related increase in sleeping problems suggests that this population should be cautious with intake. Since the use of sleeping tablets is not without risk, it seems sensible advice for people complaining of insomnia to restrict the use of caffeine-containing drinks, food, and medication, and to avoid these for several hours before bedtime.

References

1. Hughes, J.R. and Oliveto, A.H., A systematic survey of caffeine intake in Vermont, *Exp. Clin. Psychopharmacol.*, 5, 393–398, 1997.
2. Lloyd, T., Rollings, N., Eggli, D.F., Kieselhorst, K., and Chinchilli, V.M., Dietary caffeine intake and bone status of post menopausal women, *Am. J. Clin. Nutr.*, 65, 1826–1830, 1997.
3. Talcott, G.W., Poston, W.S., and Haddock, C.K., Co-occurrent use of cigarettes, alcohol, and caffeine in a retired military population, *Mil. Med.*, 163, 133–138, 1998.
4. Soroko, S., Chang, J., and Barrett-Connor, E., Reasons for changing caffeinated coffee consumption: the Rancho Bernardo study, *J. Am. Coll. Nutr.*, 15, 97–101, 1996.
5. Benowitz, N.L., Clinical pharmacology of caffeine, *Annu. Rev. Med.*, 41, 277–288, 1990.
6. Denaro, C.P., Benowitz, N.L., Brown, C.R., Wilson, M., and Jacob, P., Dose dependency of caffeine metabolism with repeated dosing, *Clin. Pharmacol. Ther.*, 48, 277–285, 1990.
7. Schnegg, M. and Lauterburg, B.H., Quantitative liver function in the elderly assessed by galactose elimination capacity, aminopyrine demethylation and caffeine clearance, *J. Hepatol.*, 3, 164–171, 1986.

8. Joeres, R., Klinker, H., Heusler, H., Epping, J., Zilly, W., and Richter, E., Influence of smoking on caffeine elimination in healthy volunteers and in patients with alcoholic liver cirrhosis, *Hepatology*, 8, 575–579, 1988.

9. Dunwiddie, T.V., The physiological role of adenosine in the central nervous system, *Int. Rev. Neurobiol.*, 27, 63–139, 1985.

10. Lader, M.H. and Bruce, M.S., The human pharmacology of the methylxanthines, in *Human Psychopharmacology; Measures and Methods*, Vol. 2, Hindmarch, I. and Stonier, P.D., Eds., John Wiley & Sons, New York, 1989.

11. Greden, J.F., Anxiety or caffeinism: a diagnostic dilemma, *Am. J. Psychol.*, 131, 1089–1092, 1974.

12. Oliveto, A.H., Hughes, J.R., Higgins, S.T., Bickel, W.K., Pepper, S.L. et al., Forced choice versus free choice procedures: caffeine self-administration in humans, *Psychopharmacology*, 109, 85–91, 1992.

13. Swift, C.G. and Tiplady, B., The effects of age on the response to caffeine, *Psychopharmacology*, 94, 29–31, 1998.

14. Arciero, P.J., Gardner, A.W., Benowitz, N.L., and Poehlman, E.T., Relationship of blood pressure, heart rate and behavioural mood state to norepinephrine kinetics in younger and older men following caffeine ingestion, *Eur. J. Clin. Nutr.*, 52, 805–812, 1998.

15. Bryant, C.A., Farmer, A., Tiplady, B., Keating, J., Sherwood, R., Swift, C.G., and Jackson, S.H., Psychomotor performance: investigating the dose–response relationship for caffeine and theophylline in elderly volunteers, *Eur. J. Clin. Pharmacol.*, 54, 309–313, 1998.

16. Rogers, P.J. and Dernoncourt, C., Regular caffeine consumption: a balance of adverse and beneficial effects for mood and psychomotor performance, *Pharmacol. Biol. Behav.*, 59, 1039–1045, 1998.

17. Buysse, D.J., Reynolds, III, C.F., Monk, T.H., Berman, S.R., and Kupfer, D.J., The Pittsburgh Sleep Quality Index: a new instrument for psychiatric practice and research, *Psychiatr. Res.*, 28, 193–213, 1988.

18. Miles, L.E. and Dement, W.C., Sleep and aging, *Sleep*, 3, 119–220, 1980.

19. Feinberg, I., Changes in sleep cycle patterns with age, *J. Psychiatr. Res.*, 10, 283–306, 1974.

20. Gillin, J.C., Duncan, W.C., Murphy, D.L. et al., Age related changes in sleep depressed and normal subjects, *Psychiatr. Res.*, 4, 73–78, 1981.

21. Bixler, E.O., Kales, A., Soldatos, C.R. et al., Prevalence of sleep disorders in the Los Angeles Metropolitan area, *Am. J. Psych.*, 136, 1257–1262, 1979.

22. Karacans, I., Thornby, J.I., Anch, M., Booth, G.H., Williams, R.L., and Salis, P.J., Dose related sleep disturbances induced by coffee and caffeine, *Clin. Pharmacol. Ther.*, 20, 682–689, 1976.

23. Colton, T., Gosselin, R.E., and Smith, R.P., The tolerance of coffee drinkers to caffeine, *Clin. Pharm. Ther.*, 199, 679–686, 1968.

24. Shirlow, M.J. and Mathers, C.D., A study of caffeine consumption and symptoms: indigestion, palpitations, tremor, headaches and insomnia, *Int. J. Epidemiol.*, 14, 239–248, 1985.

25. Morgan, K., Dallosso, H., Ebrahim, S., Arie, T., and Fentem, P.H., Characteristics of subjective insomnia in the elderly living at home, *Age Ageing*, 17, 1–7, 1988.

26. Ohayon, M.M., Caulet, M., Philip, P., Guilleminault, C., and Priest, R.G., How sleep and mental disorders are related to complaints of daytime sleepiness, *Arch. Intern. Med.*, 157, 2645–2652, 1997.

27. Morgan, K., Healey, D.W., and Healey, P.J., Factors influencing persistent subjective insomnia in old age: a follow-up study of good and poor sleepers aged 65–74, *Age Ageing*, 18, 117–122, 1989.

28. Victor, B.S., Lubetsky, M., and Greden, J.F., Somatic manifestations of caffeinism, *J. Clin. Psychiatr.*, 42, 185–188, 1981.

29. Curless, R., French, J.M., James, O.F.W., and Wynne, H.A., Is caffeine a factor in subjective insomnia of elderly people? *Age Ageing*, 22, 41–45, 1993.

30. Levy, M. and Zylber-Katz, E., Caffeine metabolism and coffee-attributed sleep disturbances, *Clin. Pharmacol. Ther.*, 33, 770–775, 1983.

31. Edelstein, B.A., Keaton-Brasted, C., and Burg, M.M., Effects of caffeine withdrawal on nocturnal enuresis, insomnia and behavior restraints, *J. Consult. Clin. Psychol.*, 52, 857–862, 1984.

32. Stephens, C.M., Hankey, C., and Wynne, H.A., Effect of caffeine-free beverages on elderly hospitalised patients, *Int. J. Pharmacol. Pract.*, 3, 245–248, 1995.

33. Brezinova, V., Effect of caffeine on sleep: EEG study in late middle age people, *Br. J. Clin. Pharmacol.*, 1, 203–208, 1974.

34. Lutz, E.G., Restless legs, anxiety and caffeinism, *J. Clin. Psychiatr.*, 39, 693–698, 1978.

35. Ancoli-Israel, S., Kripke, D.F., Mason, W.J. et al., Sleep apnea and periodic limb movements in sleep in a randomly selected elderly population: final prevalence results, *Sleep Res.*, 15, 101, 1986.

36. Ohayon, M.M., Guilleminault, C., Priest, R.G., and Caulet, M., Snoring and breathing pauses during sleep: telephone interview survey of a United Kingdom population sample, *Br. Med. J.*, 314, 860–863, 1997.

37. Okuma, T., Matsuoka, H., Matsue, Y., and Toyomura, K., Model insomnia by methylphenidate and caffeine and use in the evaluation of temazepam, *Psychopharmacology*, 76, 201–208, 1982.

38. Forrest, W.H., Bellville, J.W., and Brown, B.W., The interaction of caffeine with pentobarbital as a night time hypnotic, *Anesthesiology*, 36, 37–41, 1972.

8

Coffee and Cancer in Aging Adults

Alessandra Tavani and Carlo La Vecchia

CONTENTS

Studies on the relationship between coffee consumption and cancer risk have been mainly focused on cancers of the urinary bladder, pancreas, and colorectum, and most data refer to adult and elderly populations. The relationship between coffee and bladder cancer is controversial, although many case-control studies have been published over the last three decades. In most studies, compared to coffee nondrinkers, the odds ratio (OR) tends to be elevated in drinkers, but the excess risk is generally neither dose nor duration related. Thus, although coffee drinking may be considered a risk indicator of bladder cancer, a strong association can be excluded, and it is still unclear whether this indicator is causal or nonspecific and due to some bias or confounding. For pancreatic cancer, a possible positive association with coffee consumption was postulated in a report published in 1981; since then, however, most studies have shown no substantial association, and, thus, there is now substantial evidence that coffee is not related to pancreatic cancer risk. Overall evidence on the coffee–colorectal cancer relation suggests an inverse association: no consistent relationship was observed in five cohort studies, but most case-control studies found OR below unity for colon and close to unity for rectal cancer. A plausible biological explanation has been given in terms of reduction of bile acids and neutral sterol secretion in the colon. For other cancer sites, including oral cavity, esophagus, stomach, liver, breast, ovary, kidney, and lymphoid neoplasms, data on the relation between coffee drinking and cancer risk are limited and generally inconsistent, but largely reassuring.

Introduction

Over the last four decades, the relationship between coffee and cancer risk has been extensively investigated. Among various cancer sites considered, there are several digestive, bladder and other urinary tract, breast, genital, and lymphoid neoplasms. All the data were extensively reviewed in 1990 by a working group of the International Agency for Research of Cancer (IARC) (IARC Monograph No. 51).[1] This chapter recalls the conclusions reached by the IARC working group and extends the information to more recent findings. Since incidence of cancer at most sites increases with age, most data refer to aging adults.

Descriptive Epidemiology

Descriptive studies of temporal trends and geographic patterns (ecological studies) showed no consistent relationship between various measures of coffee consumption or disappearance and cancer rates.[1] These studies, however, are scarcely informative, as it is not possible to distinguish among coffee consumption, cigarette smoking, and alcohol drinking, which are often highly correlated.[1,2] It is not surprising, however, in view of the large number of tests performed, that some significant differences were observed, but only for pancreatic cancer the strength and consistency of the correlations reported by several studies were difficult to attribute to chance alone. Still, there are some features of the descriptive epidemiology of pancreatic cancer, such as the difficulties and uncertainties of diagnosis and certification of the disease, with the consequent higher rates in developed areas of the world and the substantial upward trends in recent decades, that may well be the explanation for the correlations. No consistent association was found between coffee consumption and bladder cancer rates in ecological and descriptive epidemiological studies.[1]

Cancer of the Bladder and Other Urinary Sites

Studies published before 1990 are summarized in the IARC Monograph No. 51[1] and by La Vecchia.[2] The IARC working group examined 26 studies, 22 of which were used to make evaluations. Of the studies, 16 showed a moderately higher risk of bladder cancer in coffee drinkers compared with nondrinkers; in seven of these the association was significant, and in three there was a dose–risk relationship. No relationship was observed in the other six studies. Lifelong nonsmokers were also considered separately, to obtain information on the impact of the potential distorting effect of tobacco: the relationship with coffee was still observed, although it was less clear, in part because of the smaller absolute numbers.[1]

Data on decaffeinated coffee from six case-control studies were reviewed, but its effect was not clearly distinguishable from that of coffee containing caffeine.[1]

After the publication of the IARC monograph, three prospective[3-5] and several case-control studies[6-14] have given information on the relation between coffee and bladder cancer. The first prospective study,[3] based on a Norwegian cohort of 43,000 men and women, found a nonsignificantly increased risk, the relative risk (RR) being 1.5 in men and 2.4 in women drinking ≥7 cups of coffee per day. The second prospective study[4] was based on 52 bladder cancers among 34,198 Californian Seventh-day Adventists who had provided information on lifestyle and dietary habits in 1976 and were followed up for six years. Compared with coffee nondrinkers, the smoking-adjusted RR was 1.0 for less than one cup per day, 0.4 for one cup, and 2.0 for two or more cups of coffee per day; the trend in risk was not significant, but the pattern was similar in smokers and nonsmokers. The third prospective study[5] was conducted on nearly 8000 Japanese-Americans living in Hawaii and included 96 incident cases diagnosed during a 22-year follow-up. High consumption of coffee increased bladder cancer risk, with no significant dose–response relationship. In a French hospital-based case-control study, based on 690 cases, Clavel and Cordier[6] found that, compared with coffee nondrinkers, the OR was 3.8 for drinkers of more then seven cups per day, with a significant trend in risk; after further allowance for smoking, the risk estimate declined to 2.9, and the trend in risk was no longer significant. In a population-based case-control study based on 261 cases of lower urinary tract cancer in both Caucasians and Japanese living in Hawaii,[7] there was no overall association with coffee drinking. In a German hospital-based case-control study of 675 cases of bladder cancer,[8] a significant twofold or more increase in risk was found for heavy consumption of coffee in both sexes after controlling for smoking. A hospital-based case-control study from Italy,[9] based on 555 cases, found an OR of 1.3 in drinkers compared with nondrinkers and of 1.4 for drinkers of four or more cups per day with a significant trend in risk when nondrinkers were included in the trend analysis; the risk was higher in people who never smoked, but there was no trend in risk with dose. In an American population-based study,[10] based on 351 bladder cancer cases, coffee consumption was associated with an increased risk of bladder cancer among the heaviest coffee drinkers (OR 2.1, significant) after adjustment for cigarette smoking and dietary factors. A multicenter population-based case-control study, conducted in Spain on 497 cases,[11] did not find any association between coffee consumption and bladder cancer risk in either sex; nonsignificantly increased risks were found in nonsmokers (OR 2.78) with a dose–response relationship for lifelong consumption and years of exposure to regular coffee. An American population-based case-control study,[12] based on 262 cases, found no association with coffee consumption and an insignificantly increased risk with decaffeinated coffee only in women. Another Italian hospital-based case-control study,[13] based on 172 cases, found a significantly increased risk in coffee drinkers (OR 2.6 in men, with a significant trend in risk with dose, and 5.2 in women), after allowance for several covariants including cigarette smoking. A hospital-based case-control study conducted in Germany on 300 cases of lower urinary tract cancer[14] found increased risk of cancer at the highest levels of coffee consumption, but the risk estimates were drastically reduced after allowance for smoking.

Thus, the results of the more recent studies on bladder cancer are consistent with previous data on the coffee–bladder cancer relationship. In biological terms, caffeine and the large number of substances other than caffeine contained in coffee have a wide spectrum of direct and indirect metabolic activities; it is conceivable that even small amounts of coffee may bring about changes in the levels of carcinogens or anticarcinogens in the bladder epithelium, since most substances or metabolites are secreted through the urinary tract and are consequently in direct contact with the bladder mucosa.[1] However, the overall epidemiological evidence allows one to exclude strong associations between coffee and bladder cancer, while suggesting that coffee drinking represents a weak indicator for bladder cancer risk. Whether this indicator is nonspecific or includes some aspects of causality is still not clear. An important confounding factor is cigarette smoking, which is related to both coffee consumption and bladder cancer risk. The difference between crude and adjusted OR varies from one study to another and misclassification of smoking status is unlikely to explain totally the positive results for all the studies. Other possible residual confounding factors might include diet or occupational exposure, although the similar associations found in males and females suggest that occupational exposures cannot totally account for the positive results.

With reference to kidney cancer, although the data are limited, a similar pattern of risk was apparent for transitional cell cancers of the renal pelvis and ureter, whose etiology and pathogenesis are in several aspects similar to those of bladder cancer.[1]

Published data on adenocarcinoma of the kidney are scarce as well, but they do not indicate any consistent association with coffee.[1] After the IARC evaluation, a population-based case-control study,[15] conducted in the Boston metropolitan area and based on 410 cases of renal cell adenocarcinoma, found an OR of 1.4 for moderate vs. low coffee drinking and 1.2 for high vs. low intake; none of these estimates was statistically significant. No association was found in a Norwegian cohort[3] and in three case-control studies, one Italian,[16] one French,[17] and one Canadian,[18] based, respectively, on 240, 196, and 518 cases. Most information on renal cell cancer, however, comes from the International Renal Cell Cancer Study, a population-based case-control study conducted in Australia, Denmark, Sweden, and the U.S. and including 1185 cases.[19] The ORs were 0.72 in men and 2.11 (significant) in women drinking six or more cups per day, with no trend in risk. The positive finding in one gender only and the lack of a dose–response relationship argues against a causal role of coffee; possibly some confounding by a correlate of coffee consumption is responsible for the increased risks in women.

Cancer of the Pancreas

The possible association between coffee consumption and the risk of pancreatic cancer gained widespread attention when a large study published in the early 1980s showed a strong positive association.[20] The IARC monograph[1] considered 21 case-control studies which provided data on the coffee–pancreatic cancer relationship: ten found moderate positive associations, which tended, however, to be weaker after allowance for smoking; and the remaining studies found no association. When the results of various studies published before 1987 were pooled to obtain an overall risk estimate for coffee consumption,[21] there seemed to be evidence of a moderate effect. Even when the data from the study,[20] which first observed the association, were excluded from the pooled analysis, the RR was 1.2 (95% confidence interval, CI, 1.0 to 1.5) for moderate drinkers and 1.4 (95% CI, 1.1 to 1.8) for heavy drinkers compared with nondrinkers. The working group recognized a modest association between elevated coffee consumption and pancreatic cancer, which might not be causal, but rather reflects bias or confounding.[1,2] Data on decaffeinated coffee were scanty and overall considered negative.[1,2]

Since then, the results of at least four cohort studies have been published.[3,22-24] No association emerged in the Norwegian cohort[3] of men and women, in a cohort of American men followed up for 20 years,[22] and in a cohort of nearly 14,000 residents of a retirement community followed up for 9 years.[23] Conversely, in the cohort of Iowa women,[24] based on 66 incident cases of pancreatic cancer, there was a statistically significant twofold elevated risk for those who drank >17.5 cups of coffee per week; the association was still positive but attenuated (p trend = 0.17) in never smokers. Most case-control studies[25-34] published after the IARC monograph found no significant association between coffee intake and pancreatic cancer risk. Only two studies[35,36] found positive association: one American study, based on 149 cases,[35] found an OR of 2.38, with similar estimates in smokers and nonsmokers and higher risk for users of decaffeinated coffee; and the other, an Italian study based on 570 cases,[36] found a statistically significant dose–response relationship, with an OR of 2.53 for consumption of more than three cups per day. It is possible, however, that this association is not causal, but explainable through residual confounding with cigarette smoking (the single recognized risk factor for pancreatic cancer)[37] or other sources of bias.

Thus, a strong association between coffee and pancreatic cancer can now be excluded, but, although the majority of the studies are largely or completely reassuring, it is not possible to totally exclude some small association.

Cancer of the Colon and Rectum

In the IARC monograph[1] the four cohort studies that addressed the issue of coffee drinking and risk of colorectal cancer have generally been interpreted as showing no association. Of the 12 informative case-control studies, 11 indicated inverse associations, which reached significance in 5; in 1 study a significant dose–response relation was observed and 1 study showed a protective effect of high levels of coffee consumpion. Thus, the IARC monograph concluded that, although bias and confounding could not be excluded, overall evidence was compatible with a protective effect of coffee on colorectal cancer.[1]

Since then, several studies have been published. A study of a Finnish clinical trial cohort,[38] based on 106 cases of colon and 79 cases of rectal cancer, and a cohort study of 43,000 Norwegian men and women,[3] based on 120 cases of colon and 69 rectal cancer cases, found no association of coffee intake with risk of cancer at either site.

Among case-control studies, a relatively small investigation of a selected population (Utah Mormons)[39] with low coffee intake found an elevated risk in men (RR 2.0, 95% CI, 1.0 to 4.2), but not in women with high coffee intake. This is not surprising, considering the peculiar correlates that may influence coffee consumption in that peculiar population. In another small study,[40] based on 49 cases of colorectal cancer, there was no relation with coffee consumption, the OR being 1.1 for drinkers of ≥8 cups per day. A protection for colorectal cancer (119 cases) was found in an Italian study,[41] with an OR of 0.38 (95% CI, 0.16 to 0.89) for more than two cups of coffee per day, and in a Swiss study[42] (OR 0.44). The inverse association was observed in various age groups, including elderly people. Conversely, a study from Argentina,[43] based on 190 cases, found no association, and a French study,[44] based on 171 cases, found no association in women and increased risk of colorectal cancer in men. A meta-analysis of coffee consumption and risk of colorectal cancer[45] published in 1998 found an RR of 0.72 (95% CI, 0.61 to 0.84) for high vs. low category of coffee consumption combining the results of 12 case-control studies, an RR of 0.97 combining the results of five cohort studies, and an RR of 0.76 (95% CI, 0.66 to 0.89) combining all studies; it concluded that although overall results suggest an inverse relation between coffee consumption and colorectal cancer risk, the results are inconclusive because of inconsistencies between cohort and case-control studies.

When colon and rectal cancer were considered separately, a Swedish study,[46] based on 352 cases, found a protective effect of coffee on colon cancer risk, with an OR 0.48 (95% CI, 0.27 to 0.86) in drinkers of ≥6 cups per day, but no association with rectal cancer (217 cases). Similarly, an Italian study,[47] based on 2166 cases of colon and 1364 cases of rectal cancer, found reduced risk of colon cancer in coffee drinkers, with an OR of 0.73 (95% CI, 0.60 to 0.89) in drinkers of ≥4 cups per day, with a significant trend with dose, and no association with rectal cancer risk. No association with colon cancer was found in an American study,[48] based on 424 cases, while another American study,[49] based on 1993 cases, found that, in men, compared with nonconsumers, low levels of coffee intake were associated with an increased risk of colon cancer (OR 1.30), while at high levels of consumption there was a reduced risk (OR 0.79, 95% CI, 0.57 to 1.09). Thus, most case-control studies suggest some inverse association between coffee consumption and cancer of the colon, but no consistent association with cancer of the rectum. A biological interpretation of the potential protection of coffee against large intestine cancer has been given in terms of a reduction of bile acid and neutral sterol secretion in the colon by substances in coffee, since bile acids are potent promoters of colon carcinogenesis in animals.[50-52]

Cancer of the Stomach and Upper Aerodigestive Tract

Data on coffee and gastric cancer risk from five case-control studies were reviewed by the IARC monograph.[1] There was no evidence of association in any of them. Since then, in the Norwegian cohort[3] there was no association between coffee intake and gastric cancer risk, while a cohort study of Japanese residents in Hawaii,[53] based on 108 cases of gastric cancer, found that, compared with nondrinkers, men who drank one cup of coffee per day had a significantly elevated risk of gastric cancer (relative hazard 2.5, 95% CI, 1.0 to 6.1). Case-control studies from several populations[54-57] found no association of coffee drinking with gastric cancer risk. Thus, evidence from published studies based on different populations indicates that coffee is unlikely to have any major impact on gastric carcinogenesis, while it certainly has an impact on gastric secretion. Six studies providing data on cancers of the oral cavity, pharynx, and esophagus were considered in the IARC monograph.[1]

There was no evidence of an association with coffee consumption in any of them, except for a possible association with very high temperature. At least five more studies have found no association of cancer of the upper aerodigestive tract,[3,58-61] while a case-control study based on 598 cases of oral and pharyngeal car ˜er[62] found that risk approximately halved in the highest compared with the lowest quintile of coffee intake.

As for gallbladder cancer risk, a case-control study[63] found no association, while another[64] found lower risks in coffee drinkers (OR 0.26, 95% CI, 0.07 to 0.95).

Cancer of the Breast

Seven case-control studies were considered in the IARC monograph and none of them found an association between breast cancer risk and coffee consumption.[1] After the IARC monograph was published, three cohort[3,65,66] and four case-control[67-70] studies — including an Italian one with nearly 6000 women with breast cancer[70] — found no association; one case-control study showed a protection in postmenopausal women.[71] Moreover, there is no reason to believe that a measurement error or confounding may be responsible for the finding.[2]

Cancer of the Ovary

At the time of the IARC monograph seven case-control studies of ovarian cancer included data on coffee: risks were significantly elevated in two of them, and a slightly increased risk was found in the remaining five.[1]

Since then, in a Norwegian cohort study[3] there was a nonstatistically significant increase in risk (RR 2.0 for ≥7 cups per day), and a hospital-based case-control study from Greater Athens,[72] based on 189 women, found no consistent association of coffee intake with ovarian cancer risk. Now the overall interpretation of the findings allows the exclusion of any appreciable association between coffee intake and ovarian cancer risk.

Cancer at Other Sites

One case-control study of cancer of the liver, two cohort and one case-control study of lung cancer, and a cohort study on Hodgkin's disease, non-Hodgkin's lymphomas, lymphatic and myeloid leukemia, and malignant melanoma were considered in the IARC monograph and found no association with coffee consumption.[1] Some association with coffee was found in a case-control study of vulvar cancer and in a cohort study of cervical cancer.[1]

More information since then has been published, further supporting the lack of association of coffee drinking with cancer of the lung[73] (except for an increase in men, but not in women in a Norwegian cohort),[3] non-Hodgkin's lymphomas,[3,74,75] Hodgkin's disease,[3,75] myelomas,[75] and soft tissue sarcomas.[75] Conversely, coffee drinking in women was associated with significant decreased risk of cutaneous malignant melanoma in a cohort of Norwegian men and women.[76] The association of coffee consumption with vulvar cancer found in the previous study[1] was confirmed in a case-control study,[77] based on 201 cases, which found that risk increased irregularly with the number of cups of coffee, so the issue is still unclear. No association with coffee intake was found in a cohort[3] and in a case-control study of endometrial cancer,[78] and in a cohort[3] and four case-control studies of prostate cancer.[79-82] An inverse association of borderline significance (OR 0.7 in the highest tertile of intake compared with the lowest) was found in a case-control study of thyroid cancer.[83]

Summary and Conclusions

This updated overview of coffee and cancer epidemiology provides further reassuring information on the absence of any appreciable association of coffee intake with most common cancers, including cancer of the genital tract, digestive tract, and breast. Most recent studies on bladder cancer exclude a strong association with coffee intake; the inconsistent findings in the two sexes in several studies, the lack of dose–response relationships, and the same findings for different types of coffee (in terms of caffeine content) do not support the hypothesis of causality. Possibly, the modest association for drinkers may depend on the residual confounding.

For pancreatic cancer, three cohort studies found no association and one, a small association attenuated in those who never smoked; among case-control studies, most found no association. Thus, a strong association between coffee intake and pancreatic cancer risk can be excluded; a modest positive association is still plausible, although it may be partly due to residual confounding of smoking.

As for colorectal cancer, four cohort studies reported no association of coffee intake with risk. Conversely, most case-control studies reported an inverse association of coffee intake with the risk of colon cancer and no association with the risk of rectal cancer. Because of the inconsistencies between cohort and case-control studies, the issue remains open.

As for other cancer sites, evidence published after the IARC working group evaluation found no strong association of coffee intake with neoplasms of the stomach, upper aerodigestive tract, breast, ovary, vulva, endometrium, prostate, lung, thyroid, non-Hodgkin's lymphoma, Hodgkin's disease, myelomas, soft tissue sarcomas, and melanomas.

Acknowledgments

This work was supported by a contribution of the Italian Association for Research on Cancer, Milan, Italy. The authors wish to thank Mrs. Judy Baggott, Ms. M. Paola Bonifacino, and the G.A. Pfeiffer Memorial Library staff for editorial assistance.

References

1. World Health Organization, *IARC Monograph Eval. Carcinog. Risk Hum.*, Geneva WHO, Vol. 51, 1991.
2. La Vecchia, C., Coffee and cancer epidemiology, in *Caffeine, Coffee, and Health*, Garattini, S., Ed., Raven Press, New York, 1993, 379.
3. Stensvold, I. and Jacobsen, B.K., Coffee and cancer: a prospective study of 43,000 Norwegian men and women, *Cancer Causes Control*, 5, 401, 1994.
4. Mills, P.K., Beeson, W.L., Phillips, R.L., and Fraser, G.E., Bladder cancer in a low risk population: results from the Adventist Health Study, *Am. J. Epidemiol.*, 133, 230, 1991.
5. Chyou, P.–H., Nomura, A.My., and Stemmermann, G.N., A prospective study of diet, smoking, and lower urinary tract cancer, *Ann. Epidemiol.*, 3, 211, 1993.
6. Clavel, J. and Cordier, S., Coffee consumption and bladder cancer risk, *Int. J. Cancer*, 47, 207, 1991.
7. Nomura, A.My., Kolonel, L.N., Hankin, J.H., and Yoshizawa, C.N., Dietary factors in cancer of the lower urinary tract, *Int. J. Cancer*, 48, 199, 1991.
8. Kunze, E., Chang-Claude, J., and Frentzel-Beyme, R., Life style and occupational risk factors for bladder cancer in Germany. A case-control study, *Cancer*, 69, 1776, 1992.
9. D'Avanzo, B., La Vecchia, C., Franceschi, S., Negri, E., Talamini, R., and Buttino, I., Coffee consumption and bladder cancer risk, *Eur. J. Cancer*, 28A, 1480, 1992.
10. Vena, J.E., Freudenheim, J., Graham, S., Marshall, J., Zielezny, M., Swanson, M., and Sufrin, G., Coffee, cigarette smoking, and bladder cancer in western New York, *Ann. Epidemiol.*, 3, 586, 1993.
11. Escolar Pujolar, A., Gonzalez, C.A., Lopez-Abente, G., Errezola, M., Izarzugaza, I., Nebot M., and Riboli, E., Bladder cancer and coffee consumption in smokers and non-smokers in Spain, *Int. J. Epidemiol.*, 22, 38, 1993.

12. Bruemmer, B., White, E., Vaughan, T.L., and Cheney, C.L., Fluid intake and the incidence of bladder cancer among middle-aged men and women in a three-county area of western Washington, *Nutr. Cancer*, 29, 163, 1997.

13. Donato, F., Boffetta, P., Fazioli R., Aulenti, V., Gelatti, U., and Porru, S., Bladder cancer, tobacco smoking, coffee and alcohol drinking in Brescia, northern Italy, *Eur. J. Epidemiol.*, 13, 795, 1997.

14. Pohlabeln, H., Jockel, K.–H., and Bolm-Audorff, U., Non-occupational risk factors for cancer of the lower urinary tract in Germany, *Eur. J. Epidemiol.*, 15, 411, 1999.

15. Maclure, M. and Willett, W., A case-control study of diet and risk of renal adenocarcinoma, *Epidemiology*, 1, 430, 1990.

16. Talamini, R., Baron, A.E., Barra, S., Bidoli, E., La Vecchia, C., Negri, E., Serraino, D., and Franceschi, S., A case-control study of risk factor for renal cell cancer in northern Italy, *Cancer Causes Control*, 1, 125, 1990.

17. Benhamou, S., Lenfant, M.H., Ory-Paoletti, C., and Flamant, R., Risk factors for renal-cell carcinoma in a French case-control study, *Int. J. Cancer*, 55, 32, 1993.

18. Kreiger, N., Marrett, L.D., Dodds, L., Hilditch, S., and Darlington, G.A., Risk factors for renal cell carcinoma: results of a population-based case-control study, *Cancer Causes Control*, 4, 101, 1993.

19. Wolk, A., Gridley, G., Niwa, S., Lindblad, P., McCredie, M., Mellemgaard, A., Mandel, J.S., Wahrendorf, J., McLaughlin, J.K., and Adami, H.-O., International renal cell cancer study. VII. Role of diet, *Int. J. Cancer*, 65, 67, 1996.

20. MacMahon, B., Yen, S., Trichopoulos, D., Warren, K., and Nardi, G., Coffee and cancer of the pancreas, *N. Engl. J. Med.*, 304, 630, 1981.

21. La Vecchia, C., Liati, P., Decarli, A., Negri, E., and Franceschi, S., Coffee consumption and risk of pancreatic cancer, *Int. J. Cancer*, 40, 309, 1987.

22. Zheng, W., McLaughlin, J.K., Gridley, G., Bjelke, E., Schuman, L.M., Silverman, D.T., Wacholder, S., Co-Chien, H.T., Blot, W.J., and Fraumeni, J.F., Jr., A cohort study of smoking, alcohol consumption, and dietary factors for pancreatic cancer (United States), *Cancer Causes Control*, 4, 477, 1993.

23. Shibata, A., Mack, T.M., Paganini-Hill, A., Ross, R.K., and Henderson, B.E., A prospective study of pancreatic cancer in the elderly, *Int. J. Cancer*, 58, 46, 1994.

24. Harnack, L.J., Anderson, K.E., Zheng, W., Folsom, A.R., Sellers, T.A., and Kushi, L.H., Smoking, alcohol, coffee, and tea intake and incidence of cancer of exocrine pancreas: the Iowa Women's Health Study, *Cancer Epidemiol. Biomarkers Prev.*, 6, 1081, 1997.

25. Farrow, D.C. and Davis, S., Risk of pancreatic cancer in relation to medical history and the use of tobacco, alcohol and coffee, *Int. J. Cancer*, 45, 816, 1990.

26. Baghurst, P.A., McMichael, A.J., Slavotinek, A.H., Baghurst, K.J., Boyle, P., and Walker, A.M., A case-control study of diet and cancer of the pancreas, *Am. J. Epidemiol.*, 134, 167, 1991.

27. Ghadirian, P., Simard, A., and Baillargeon, J., Tobacco, alcohol, and coffee and cancer of the pancreas. A population-based case-conrol study in Quebec, Canada, *Cancer*, 67, 2664, 1991.

28. Jain, M., Howe, G.R., St. Louis, P., and Miller, A.B., Coffee and alcohol as determinants of risk of pancreas cancer: a case-control study from Toronto, *Int. J. Cancer*, 47, 384, 1991.

29. Bueno de Mesquita, H.B., Maisonneuve, P., Moerman, C.J., Runia, S., and Boyle, P., Lifetime consumption of alcoholic beverages, tea and coffee and exocrine carcinoma of the pancreas: a population-based case-control study in the Netherlands, *Int. J. Cancer*, 50, 514, 1992.

30. Friedman, G.D. and van den Eeden, S.K., Risk factors for pancreatic cancer: an exploratory study, *Int. J. Epidemiol.*, 22, 30, 1993.

31. Kalapothaki, V., Tznou, A., Hsieh, C.C., Toupadaki, N., Karakatsani, A., and Trichopoulos, D., Tobacco, ethanol, coffee, pancreatitis, diabetes mellitus, and cholelithiasis as risk factors for pancreatic carcinoma, *Cancer Causes Control*, 4, 375, 1993.

32. Zatonski, W.A., Boyle, P., Przewozniak, K., Maisonneuve, P., Drosik, K., and Walker, A.M., Cigarette smoking, alcohol, tea and coffee consumption and pancreas cancer risk: a case-control study from Opole, Poland, *Int. J. Cancer*, 53, 601, 1993.

33. Partanen, T., Hemminki, K., Vainio, H., and Kauppinen, T., Coffee consumption not associated with risk of pancreas cancer in Finland, *Prev. Med.*, 24, 213, 1995.

34. Soler, M., Chatenoud, L., La Vecchia, C., Franceschi, S., and Negri, E., Diet, alcohol, coffee and pancreatic cancer: final results from an Italian study, *Eur. J. Cancer Prev.*, 7, 455, 1998.

35. Lyon, J.L., Mahoney, A.W., French, T.K., and Moser, R., Jr., Coffee consumption and the risk of cancer of the exocrine pancreas: a case-control study in a low-risk population, *Epidemiology*, 3, 164, 1992.

36. Gullo, L., Pezzilli, R., and Morselli-Labate, A.M., Coffee and cancer of the pancreas: an Italian multicenter study. The Italian Pancreatic Cancer Study Group, *Pancreas*, 11, 223, 1995.

37. Boyle, P., Hsieh, C.C., Maisonneuve, P., La Vecchia, C., Macfarlane, G.J., Walker, A.M., and Trichopoulos, D., Epidemiology of pancreas cancer (1988), *Int. J. Pancreatol.*, 5, 327, 1989.

38. Hartman, T.J., Tangrea, J.A., Pietinen, P., Malila, N., Virtanen, M., Taylor, P.R., and Albanes, D., Tea and coffee consumption and risk of colon and rectal cancer in middle-aged Finnish men, *Nutr. Cancer*, 31, 41, 1998.

39. Slattery, M.L., West, D.W., Robinson L.M., French, T.K., Ford, M.H., Schuman, K.L., and Sorenson, A.W., Tobacco, alcohol, coffee, and caffeine as risk factors for colon cancer in a low-risk population, *Epidemiology*, 1, 141, 1990.

40. Olsen, J. and Kronborg, O., Coffee, tobacco and alcohol as risk factors for cancer and adenoma of the large intestine, *Int. J. Epidemiol.*, 22, 398, 1993.

41. Centonze, S., Boeing, H., Leoci, C., Guerra, V., and Misciagna, G., Dietary habits and colorectal cancer in a low-risk area. Results from a population-based case-control study in southern Italy, *Nutr. Cancer*, 21, 233, 1994.

42. Levi, F., Pasche, C., La Vecchia, C., Lucchini, F., and Franceschi S., Food groups and colorectal cancer risk, *Br. J. Cancer*, 79, 1283, 1999.

43. Muñoz, S.E., Navarro, A., Lantieri, M.J., Fabro, M.E., Peyrano, M.G., Ferraroni, M., Decarli A., La Vecchia, C., and Eynard, A.R., Alcohol, methylxanthine-containing beverages, and colorectal cancer in Cordoba, Argentina, *Eur. J. Cancer Prev.*, 7, 207, 1998.

44. Boutron-Ruault, M.C., Senesse, P., Faivre, J., Chatelain, N., Belghiti, C., and Meance, S., Foods as risk factors for colorectal cancer: a case-control study in Burgundy (France), *Eur. J. Cancer Prev.*, 8, 229, 1999.

45. Giovannucci, E., Meta-analysis of coffee consumption and risk of colorectal cancer, *Am. J. Epidemiol.*, 147, 1043, 1998.

46. Baron, J.A., Gerhardsson de Verdier, M., and Ekbom, A., Coffee, tea, tobacco, and cancer of the large bowel, *Cancer Epidemiol. Biomarkers Prev.*, 3, 565, 1994.
47. Tavani, A., Pregnolato, A., La Vecchia, C., Negri, E., Talamini, R., and Franceschi, S., Coffee and tea intake and risk of cancers of the colon and rectum: a study of 3,530 cases and 7,057 controls, *Int. J. Cancer*, 73, 193, 1997.
48. Shannon, J., White, E., Shattuck, A.L., and Potter, J.D., Relationship of food groups and water intake to colon cancer risk, *Cancer Epidemiol. Biomarkers Prev.*, 5, 495, 1996.
49. Slattery, M.L., Caan, B.J., Anderson, K.E., and Potter, J.D., Intake of fluids and methylxanthine-containing beverages: association with colon cancer, *Int. J. Cancer*, 81, 199, 1999.
50. La Vecchia, C., Epidemiological evidence on coffee and digestive tract cancers: a review, *Digestive Dis.*, 8, 281, 1990.
51. Bjelke, E., Colon cancer and blood cholesterol, *Lancet*, 1, 1116, 1974.
52. Jacobsen, B.K. and Thelle, D.S., Coffee, cholesterol, and colon cancer: is there a link? *Br. Med. J.*, 294, 4, 1987.
53. Galanis, D.J., Kolonel, L.N., Lee, J., and Nomura, A., Intakes of selected foods and beverages and the incidence of gastric cancer among the Japanese residents of Hawaii: a prospective study, *Int. J. Epidemiol.*, 27, 173, 1998.
54. Agudo, A., Gonzalez, C.A., Marcos, G., Sanz, M., Saigi, E., Verge, J., Boleda, M., and Ortego, J., Consumption of alcohol, coffee, and tobacco, and gastric cancer in Spain, *Cancer Causes Control*, 3, 137, 1992.
55. Hansson, L.E., Nyren, O., Bergstrom, R., Wolk, A., Lindgren, A., Baron, J., and Adami, H.–O., Diet and risk of gastric cancer. A population-based case-control study in Sweden, *Int. J. Cancer*, 55, 181, 1993.
56. Chow, W.H., Swanson, C.A., Lissowska, J., Groves, F.D., Sobin, L.H., Nasierowska-Guttmejer, A., Radziszewski, J., Regula, J., Hsing, A.W., Jagannatha, S., Zantonski, W., and Blot, W.J., Risk of stomach cancer in relation to consumption of cigarettes, alcohol, tea and coffee in Warsaw, Poland, *Int. J. Cancer*, 81, 871, 1999.
57. Inoue, M., Tajima, K., Hirose, K., Hamajima, N., Takezaki, T., Kuroishi, T., and Tominaga, S., Tea and coffee consumption and the risk of digestive tract cancers: data from a comparative case-referent study in Japan, *Cancer Causes Control*, 9, 209, 1998.
58. La Vecchia, C., Negri, E., D'Avanzo, B., Franceschi, S., Decarli, A., and Boyle, P., Dietary indicators of laryngeal cancer risk, *Cancer Res.*, 50, 4497, 1990.
59. Franceschi, S., Bidoli, E., Baron, A.E., Barra, S., Talamini, R., Serraino, D., and La Vecchia, C., Nutrition and cancer of the oral cavity and pharynx in North-East Italy, *Int. J. Cancer*, 47, 20, 1991.
60. Pintos, J., Franco, E.L., Oliveira, B.V., Kowalski, L.P., Curado, M.P., and Dewar, R., Mate, coffee, and tea consumption and risk of cancers of the upper aerodigestive tract in southern Brazil, *Epidemiology*, 5, 583, 1994.
61. Bundgaard, T., Wildt, J., Frydenberg, M., Elbrond, O., and Nielsen, J.E., Case-control study of squamous cell cancer of the oral cavity in Denmark, *Cancer Causes Control*, 6, 57, 1995.
62. Franceschi, S., Favero, A., Conti, E., Talamini, R., Volpe, R., Negri, E., Barzan, L., and La Vecchia, C., Food groups, oils and butter, and cancer of the oral cavity and pharynx, *Br. J. Cancer*, 80, 614, 1999.

63. Zatonski, W.A., La Vecchia, C., Przewozniak, K., Maisonneuve, P., Lowenfels, A.B., and Boyle, P., Risk factors of gallbladder cancer: a Polish case-control study, *Int. J. Cancer*, 51, 707, 1992.

64. Ghadirian, P., Simard, A., and Baillargeon, J., A population-based case-control study of cancer of the bile ducts and gallbladder in Quebec, Canada, *Rev. Epidemiol. Sante Publique*, 41, 107, 1993.

65. Hunter, D.J., Manson, J.E., Stampfer, M.J., Colditz, G.A., Rosner, B., Hennekens, C.H., Speizer, F.E., and Willett, W.C., A prospective study of caffeine, coffee, tea, and breast cancer, *Am. J. Epidemiol.*, 136, 1000, 1992.

66. Folsom, A.R., McKenzie, D.R., Bisgard, K.M., Kushi, L.H., and Sellers, T.A., No association between caffeine intake and postmenopausal breast cancer incidence in the Iowa Women's Health Study, *Am. J. Epidemiol.*, 138, 380, 1993.

67. McLaughlin, C.C., Mahoney, M.C., Nasca, P.C., Metzger, B.B., Baptiste, M.S., and Field, N.A., Breast cancer and methylxanthine consumption, *Cancer Causes Control*, 3, 175, 1992.

68. Levi, F., La Vecchia, C., Gulie, C., and Negri, E., Dietary factors and breast cancer risk in Vaud, Switzerland, *Nutr. Cancer*, 19, 327, 1993.

69. Smith, S.J., Deacon, J.M., and Chilvers, C.E., Alcohol, smoking, passive smoking and caffeine in relation to breast cancer risk in young women. UK National Case-Control Study Group, *Br. J. Cancer*, 70, 112, 1994.

70. Tavani, A., Pregnolato, A., La Vecchia, C., Favero, A., and Franceschi, S., Coffee consumption and the risk of breast cancer, *Eur. J. Cancer Prev.*, 7, 77, 1998.

71. Mannisto, S., Pietinen, P., Virtanen, M., Kataja, V., and Uusitupa, M., Diet and risk of breast cancer in a case-control study: does the threat of disease have an influence on recall bias? *J. Clin. Epidemiol.*, 52, 429, 1999.

72. Polychronopoulou, A., Tzonou, A., Hsieh, C.C., Kaprinis, G., Rebelakos, A., Toupadaki, N., and Trichopoulos, D., Reproductive variables, tobacco, ethanol, coffee and somatometry as risk factors for ovarian cancer, *Int. J. Cancer*, 55, 402, 1993.

73. Mendilaharsu, M., De Stefani, E., Deneo-Pellegrini, H., Carzoglio, J.C., and Ronco, A., Consumption of tea and coffee and the risk of lung cancer in cigarette-smoking men: a case-control study in Uruguay, *Lung Cancer*, 19, 101, 1998.

74. Tavani, A., Negri, E., Franceschi, S., Talamini, R., and La Vecchia, C., Coffee consumption and risk of non-Hodgkin's lymphoma, *Eur. J. Cancer Prev.*, 3, 351, 1994.

75. Tavani, A., Pregnolato, A., Negri, E., Franceschi, S., Serraino, D., Carbone, A., and La Vecchia, C., Diet and risk of lymphoid neoplasms and soft tissue sarcomas, *Nutr. Cancer*, 27, 256, 1997.

76. Veierod, M.B., Thelle, D.S., and Laake, P., Diet and risk of cutaneous malignant melanoma: a prospective study of 50,757 Norwegian men and women, *Int. J. Cancer*, 71, 600, 1997.

77. Sturgeon, S.R., Ziegler, R.G., Brinton, L.A., Nasca, P.C., Mallin, K., and Gridley, G., Diet and the risk of vulvar cancer, *Ann. Epidemiol.*, 1, 427, 1991.

78. Levi, F., Franceschi, S., Negri, E., and La Vecchia, C., Dietary factors and the risk of endometrial cancer, *Cancer*, 71, 3575, 1993.

79. Talamini, R., Franceschi, S., La Vecchia, C., Serraino, D., Barra, S., and Negri, E., Diet and prostatic cancer: a case-control study in Northern Italy, *Nutr. Cancer*, 18, 277, 1992.

80. Slattery, M.L. and West, D.W., Smoking, alcohol, coffee, tea, caffeine and theo-bromine: risk of prostate cancer in Utah (United States), *Cancer Causes Control*, 4, 559, 1993.

81. Jain, M.G., Hislop, G.T., Howe, G.R., Burch, J.D., and Ghadirian, P., Alcohol and other beverage use and prostate cancer risk among Canadian men, *Int. J. Cancer*, 78, 707, 1998.

82. Hsieh, C.C., Thanos, A., Mitropoulos, D., Deliveliotis, C., Mantzoros, C.S., and Trichopoulos, D., Risk factors for prostate cancer: a case-control study in Greece, *Int. J. Cancer*, 80, 699, 1999.

83. Franceschi, S., Levi, F., Negri, E., Fassina, A., and La Vecchia, C., Diet and thyroid cancer: a pooled analysis of four European case-control studies, *Int. J. Cancer*, 48, 395, 1991.

9

Alcohol and Tobacco Abuse, and the Health of Aging People

Jin Zhang and Ronald R. Watson

CONTENTS

Introduction

The size of the elderly population in the U.S. has grown substantially during the 20th century and is projected to rise well into the next century. Life expectancy has continued to rise for Americans and is now over 75 years.[1] This portion of the population is expected to have a significant impact on national use of social and health services, primarily in the area of aging-related cardiovascular disease and cancer.[2]

Alcohol-related problems are often unrecognized in the elderly population. Although it is true that the prevalence of alcohol problems decreases with increasing age in the population, among older individuals who drink, the proportion of heavy drinkers is just as high as among younger age groups.[3] As a matter of fact, the rates of alcohol abuse declined with age up to age 60, began to increase for both men and women older than 60, and were particularly notable for men age 75 and older.[4] Alcohol-related illness and injury have an important impact on health in old age, and heavy drinking must be kept in the differential diagnosis of many health problems. About 15 to 20 million Americans suffer from alcohol abuse or dependence, which leads to annual losses of more than $80 billion and 100,000 lives. Approximately 21% of all the intensive care unit admissions are directly related to alcohol, and 20 to 40% of all persons admitted to general hospitals have alcohol-linked problems.[5]

Indeed, alcoholism affects virtually all organs of the body. The level and duration of alcohol consumption are important determinants of the development of liver pathology and chronic pancreatitis. Alcohol impairs or causes structural or functional changes of the mucosa of the stomach or intestine. Furthermore, alcohol affects the cardiovascular system in many different ways. Epidemiological studies demonstrated that alcohol is also strongly associated with cancer. Additional medical conditions are prevalent among alcoholics, including nutritional deficiencies (deficiencies of iron, thiamine, folate, vitamin A, and zinc).[6]

Generally, smoking rates among persons with a history of alcohol abuse are much higher than those of the general public.[7] Epidemiological evidence that light to moderate consumption of alcohol has beneficial effects on overall health, and on coronary disease in particular, is due to the increase of high-density lipoprotein (HDL) with alcohol consumption. However, a highly significant fall in HDL with smoking was observed. Smoking only 10 cigarettes or fewer per day was sufficient to negate the beneficial effect of moderate drinking on HDL.[8]

Tobacco smoking is an important cause of coronary heart disease.[9-11] It is estimated that approximately 450,000 Americans die each year from diseases directly attributable to smoking; 29% of all deaths from coronary heart disease are attributable to smoking.[12] Furthermore, tobacco smoking is a contributing factor of cancer; 38% percent of all cancer deaths in men and 23% of all cancer deaths in women are related to cigarette smoking.[13] The medical care of all smoking-related diseases cost an estimated $21.9 billion in 1993.[14]

Cardiovascular Disease

Cardiovascular disease (CVD) refers to a wide variety of heart and blood vessel diseases, including coronary heart disease (CHD), hypertension, stroke, and rheumatic heart disease. CVD is the leading cause of death and disability in the U.S.[15] Death rates for CVD markedly increase among older adults. CVD is the most common cause of death in older men. Independent risk factors for CVD in older men include increasing age, cigarette smoking, hypertension, diabetes mellitus, high serum cholesterol, and low serum HDL cholesterol.[16]

Alcohol Abuse and Cardiovascular Disease

Although considerable evidence exists that moderate drinking protects against mortality and morbidity from coronary heart disease,[17,18] heavy consumption is shown to have deleterious cardiovascular effects. It exerts its adverse effects by increasing the risks of cardiomyopathy, hypertension, and stroke.[19] Hypertension is an extremely common condition among elderly people and is a major risk factor for stroke, myocardial infarction, and other adverse vascular sequelae. There is an increased prevalence of hypertension among heavy drinkers as well as a dose–response relationship between usual alcohol use and level of systolic blood pressure.[20]

Stroke is a leading cause of death and morbidity. Hypertension, including borderline hypertension, is probably the most important stroke risk factor based on degree of risk and prevalence. However, cardiac morbidity, cigarette smoking, diabetes, physical inactivity, and high levels of alcohol consumption are also strongly related to stroke risk.[21] Alcohol may increase the risk for stroke through various mechanisms that include hypertension, hypercoagulable states, cardiac arrhythmias, and cerebral blood flow reductions.[22] Abnormalities of serum lipids, triglyceride, cholesterol, low-density lipoprotein (LDL), and HDL, are regarded as atherosclerosis risk factors.[23,24] A previous study has investigated the changes in serum lipids with smoking and drinking in a large sample of men. Both social habits were found to raise serum cholesterol levels in a dose-related manner — the more cigarettes a subject smokes and the more alcohol consumed, the higher the total serum cholesterol. Atherosclerosis (the buildup of fat and cholesterol in the arteries) is the underlying condition leading to the increased risk of death due to cardiovascular disease.[8]

Tobacco Smoking and Cardiovascular Disease

Cigarette smoking has been established as an independent determinant of stroke. In case-control and cohort studies, the effect of cigarette smoking remained significant after adjustment for other factors and a dose–response relationship was apparent.[25] Stroke risk was increased twofold in heavy smokers (more than 40 cigarettes/day) compared with light smokers (fewer than 10 cigarettes/day) and was reduced among those who quit smoking within 5 years of stroke onset compared with those who continued to smoke.[26,27]

Smoking acts in combination with other major risk factors (e.g., hypertension, elevated blood cholesterol) to increase a person's risk for CHD greatly.[28] Moreover, cigarette smoking is one of the most important risk factors for atherosclerosis. The effects of nicotine and carbon monoxide on blood vessel walls, unfavorable lipid profiles, increased myocardial work, and the decreased oxygen-carrying capacity of the blood of smokers contribute to the overall effect of cigarette smoking on cardiovascular disease (Table 9.1).[13]

TABLE 9.1

Factors Contributing to Ischemic Heart Disease among Tobacco Users

Condition	Proposed Mechanism
Atherosclerosis	Nicotine accelerates atherosclerosis; nicotine or cigarette smoke directly damages endothelium
Thrombosis	"Hypercoagulable state" from higher levels of fibrinogen and hematocrits among smokers likely related more to combustion products and gases than to nicotine; nicotine also enhances platelet aggregation
Coronary vasospasm	Possibly due to high arterial blood levels of nicotine achieved during smoking (as opposed to venous levels achieved through nicotine replacement therapy); some studies suggest, however, that nicotine is not the agent responsible for vasospasm
Arrhythmias	Nicotine stimulates catecholamine release, possibly lowering arrhythmia thresholds; catecholamines and relative polycythemia may increase myocardial oxygen demand, and in setting of stenotic coronary arteries and elevated carboxyhemoglobin levels, this may result in ischemia leading to arrhythmias
Adverse lipid profiles	Nicotine enhances lipolysis, releasing free fatty acids which results in higher LDL and lower HDL levels; smokers may also have unhealthy diets with higher fat and lower fiber and micronutrient intakes

Source: B.E. Mitchell, H.L. Sobel, and M.H. Alexander, The adverse health effects of tobacco and tobacco-related products, primary care, *Clin. Office Pract.*, 26(3), 463–498, 1999. With permission.

Of the increased cardiovascular risk caused by smoking, it is estimated that approximately one tenth of this is due to smoking-induced changes in serum lipid.[29] The majority of studies indicate elevations in serum cholesterol, phospholipids, triglycerides, and LDL and very low density lipoprotein (VLDL) cholesterol in smokers, with decreased serum HDL cholesterol.[30] In addition to its direct effect on lipids, cigarette smoking is associated with unhealthy eating patterns, including increased intakes of energy, total fat, saturated fat, cholesterol, and alcohol and lower intake of polyunsaturated fats, vitamins C and E, and beta-carotene.[31,32] These are all risk factors for cardiovascular disease.

Cancer

The causes of much of human cancer remain obscure. However, there is substantial evidence that about 80% of human cancer could be avoided by eliminating tobacco consumption; by dietary changes; and by reducing infection with certain viruses, bacteria, and parasitic worms. Alcohol behavior also contributes to the cancer burden.[33]

Alcohol Abuse and Cancer

The risk of some cancers increases among heavy drinkers. The evidence is clearest in the case of cancers of the head and neck. The risk of cancer of the mouth, pharynx, and larynx increases with consumption of more than two alcoholic drinks per day and continues to rise with increasing levels of alcohol intake.[34,35] Smoking increases this risk. It is estimated that 75% of head and neck cancers are caused by alcohol, tobacco, or both.[34,35] Among patients with head and neck cancers, mortality is higher among those who drink heavily.[36] Heavy drinking also increases the risk of esophageal cancer by fivefold or more, a risk further increased by smoking. Alcohol contributes substantially to cancer of the liver, which usually, but not always, is preceded by cirrhosis in alcoholics.[35]

Epidemiological studies show a strong association between ethanol consumption and various types of cancer.[37] Although the exact mechanisms by which chronic alcohol ingestion stimulates carcinogenesis are not known, experimental studies in animals support the concept that ethanol is not a carcinogen, but under certain experimental conditions is a cocarcinogen and/or (especially in the liver) a tumor promoter.[38] The cocarcinogenic effect of alcohol may be due to its facilitation of the actions of carcinogens by enhancing oxidant production, as well as inhibiting cell-mediated immunity (Figure 9.1). Ethanol suppresses cellular immune function and immunity particularly with short-term, high intake, or long-term, chronic intake. Ethanol consumption reduces natural killer cell function, phagocytosis, T-cell mitogenesis, and regulatory cytokine production. The metabolism of ethanol leads to the generation of acetaldehyde and free radicals[39] (Table 9.2). These highly reactive compounds bind rapidly to cell constituents and possibly to DNA. Acetaldehyde decreases DNA repair mechanisms and the methylation of cytosine in DNA. Changes in the lipid content or composition of lymphocyte membrane (vitamin E or lipid peroxide content) could stimulate or suppress the lymphoid cell functions during tumor resistance. Other mechanisms by which alcohol stimulates carcinogenesis include the induction of cytochrome P4502E1, associated with an enhanced activation of various procarcinogens present in alcoholic beverages, in association with tobacco smoke and in diets, a change in the metabolism and distribution of carcinogens, alterations in cell cycle behavior such as cell cycle duration leading to hyperregeneration. The prevalence and nature of nutritional deficiencies such as methionine, vitamin A, folate, pyridoxal phosphate, zinc, and selenium deficiencies seen in chronic alcoholics may also be associated with depressed cellular immune defenses and could function to increase cancer growth.[38]

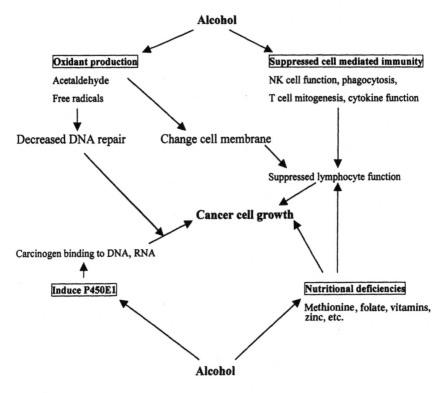

FIGURE 9.1
Alcohol and its carcinogenic mechanism.

TABLE 9.2

Metabolic and Toxic Effects of Acetaldehyde

1.	Alteration of biogenic amine metabolism
2.	Formation of proaddictive isoquinoline opioid-like substances
3.	Inhibition of mitochondrial oxidative phosphorylation
4.	Inhibition of protein synthesis
5.	Formation of adducts with thiol and amine groups in amino acids and peptides
6.	Formation of autoantibodies to acetaldehyde neoantigen adducts
7.	Generation of free radicals and reactive oxygen species
8.	Lipid peroxidation
9.	Microtubule disruption
10.	Impaired vitamin metabolism

Source: T.J. Peters and V.R. Preedy, Metabolic consequences of alcohol ingestion, *Alcohol Cardiovasc. Dis.*, 216, 19–34, 1998. With permission.

Tobacco Smoking and Cancer

Smoking is a risk factor for not only cardiovascular disease but also a variety of cancers, including lung cancer. The role of cigarette smoke and the patho-physiology of cancer are complex. Evidence found that cigarette smoke had carcinogenic potential.[40] Of some 4000 components of tobacco, more than 50 have been shown carcinogenic *in vivo* and *in vitro*.[41,42] Metabolic activation by oxidation in rat lungs creates unstable metabolites that react with DNA to form methylated bases. These methylated bases correspond to point mutations in the k-ras oncogene.[44-46] Clinically, 20 to 30% of adenocarcinoma in smokers have activated mutated k-ras oncogene.[43,47] Furthermore, elevated levels of alkylated DNA have been found in lung and trachea cells of smokers.[48]

Lung cancer is the leading cause of cancer deaths independent of sex.[49,50] Smoking was directly responsible for 83% of lung cancer deaths, or nearly one third of all cancer mortality in 1995.[51,52] The rise in lung cancer rates in men who smoke preceded the rise in women who smoke. In the early 1960s, mortality in men was approximately seven times that of women. By the late 1980s male mortality from smoking was only two and a half times that of females.[53] Currently, lung cancer rates for women approximate those for men of three decades ago.[54] Lung cancer potential from smoking has been largely attributed to polycyclic aromatic hydrocarbons (PAHs) and tobacco-specific nitrosamines (TSNAs), with a small contribution by polonium-210 and volatile aldehydes. Carcinogenicity is enhanced by cocarcinogenic catecholamines, nitrous oxides, and weakly acidic promoters. TSNAs have been shown to cause adenocarcinoma in rats, mice, and hamsters. TSNAs are organ specific. For example, 4-(methylnitrosamine)-1-(3-pyridyl)-1-butone (NNK) and 4-(methylnitrosamino)-1-(3-pyridyl)-1-butanol (NNAL) have lung carcinoma potential.[55]

Conclusions

Alcohol abuse and tobacco smoking are two major preventable causes of deaths for the aging population in the U.S. Particularly, they are both highly related to the occurrence of cardiovascular disease and cancer. In the pathogenesis of cardiovascular disease, changes in lipid metabolism related to both alcoholism and tobacco smoking play an important role. For the pathogenesis of cancer, it is a little more complicated. Although alcohol and tobacco abuse induce cancer via different mechanisms, in common they both develop free radicals. Free radical damage to cellular membranes appears to underlie alterations in function in aging and various pathological processes, including cardiovascular disease and cancer. Evidence exists for changes in membrane hydrocarbon core width and molecular volume resulting from phospholipid peroxidation, which may contribute to perturbations in membrane structure/function relationships associated with aging and cardiovascular disease.[56]

In conclusion, alcohol abuse and tobacco smoking can also cause unhealthy dietary intake, which can result in nutritional deficiency and suppressed cellular immunity. The combination adverse effect of alcohol, tobacco abuse, and unhealthy dietary patterns will predispose aging people to high risk of cardiovascular disease and cancer.

References

1. U.S. Bureau of the Census: *Statistical Abstract of the United States*, 116th ed., U.S. Government Printing Office, Washington, D.C., 1996.
2. Cobbs, E.L. and Ralapati, A.N., Health of older women, *Med. Clin. North Am.*, 82(1), 127–144, 1998.
3. Williams, Q.D. and DeBakey, S.F., Changes in levels of alcohol consumption: United States 1983–1988, *Br. J. Addict.*, 87, 643–648, 1992.
4. Eaton, W.W., Kramer, M., Anthony, J.C. et al., The incidence of specific DIS/DSM-III mental disorders. Data from the NIMH Epidemiologic Catchment Area Program, *Acta Psychiatr. Scand.*, 79, 163–178, 1989.
5. Lieber, C.S., Hepatic and other medical disorders of alcoholism: from pathogenesis to treatment, *J. Stud. Alcohol*, 59(1), 9–25, 1998.
6. Chou, S.P., Grant, B.F., and Dawson, D.A., Medical consequences of alcohol consumption — United States, 1992, *Alcohol. Clin. Exp. Res.*, 20(8), 1423–1429, 1996.
7. McIlvain, H.E., Bobo, J.K., Leed-Kelly, A., and Sitorius, M.A., Practical steps to smoking cessation for recovering alcoholics, *Am. Fam. Physician*, 57(8), 1869–1876, 1879–1882, 1998.
8. Whitehead, T.P., Robinson, D., and Allaway, S.L., The effects of cigarette smoking and alcohol consumption on blood lipids: a dose-related study on men, *Ann. Clin. Biochem.*, 33, 99–106, 1996.
9. Bartecchi, C.E., MacKenzie, T.K., and Schrier, R.W., The human cost of tobacco use, *N. Engl. J. Med.*, 330, 907–912, 975–980, 1994.
10. Rigotti, N.A. and Pasternak, R.C., Cigarette smoking and coronary heart disease: risk and management, *Cardiol. Clin.*, 14(1), 51–68, 1996.
11. U.S. Department of Health and Human Services, Reducing the Health Consequences of Smoking: 25 Years of Progress: A Report of the Surgeon General, U.S. Department of Health and Human Services, Public Health Service, Centers for Disease Control, Office on Smoking and Health, DHHS Publication No. (CDC) 89-8411, 1989.
12. Jonas, M.A., Oates, J.A., Ockene, J.K. et al., Statement on smoking and cardiovascular disease for health care professionals: AHA Medical/Scientific Statement, *Circulation*, 86, 1664–1669, 1992.

13. Mitchell, B.E., Sobel, H.L., and Alexander, M.H., The adverse health effects of tobacco and tobacco-related products, primary care, *Clin. Office Pract.*, 26(3), 463–498, 1999.
14. Centers for Disease Control and Prevention, Medical-care expenditures attributable to cigarette smoking — United States, 1993, *MMWR*, 43, 469–472, 1994.
15. Anderson, R.N., Kochonck, K.D., and Murphy, S.L., A report of final mortality statistics, *1995 Month. Vital Stat. Rep.*, 1997, 45, 11(Suppl. 2), Hyattsville, MD, National Center for Health Statistics, 1997, DHHS publication 97-1120.
16. Aronow, W.S., The older man's heart and heart disease, *Med. Clin. North Am.*, 83(5), 1291–1303, 1999.
17. Coate, D., Moderate drinking and coronary heart disease mortality: evidence from NHANES I and the NHANES I follow-up, *Am. J. Public Health*, 83, 888–890, 1993.
18. Moore, R.D. and Pearson, T.A., Moderate alcohol consumption and coronary artery disease: a review, *Medicine*, 65, 242–267, 1986.
19. Lands, W.E.M. and Zakhari, S., Alcohol use as a secondary cause of hypertension, *Mil. Med.*, 153, 250–251, 1988.
20. Adams, W.L., Alcohol and the health of aging men, *Med. Clin. North Am.*, 83(5), 1195–1210, 1999.
21. Sacco, R.L., Wolf, P.A., and Gorelick, P.B., Risk factors and their management for stroke prevention: outlook for 1999 and beyond, *Neurology*, 53(7 Suppl. 4), S15–S24, 1999.
22. Sacco, R.L., Risk factors, outcomes, and stroke subtypes for ischemic stroke, *Neurology*, 49(5), PS039–PS044, 1997.
23. Qizilbash, N., Duffy, S.W., Warlos, C., and Mann, J., Lipids are risk factors for ischemic stroke overview and review, *Cerebrovasc. Dis.*, 2, 127–136, 1992.
24. Summary of the National Cholesterol Education Program (NCEP) Adult Treatment Panel II Report, *JAMA*, 269, 3015–3023, 1993.
25. Shinton, R. and Beevers, G., Meta-analysis of relation between cigarette smoking and stroke, *Br. Med. J.*, 298, 789–794, 1989.
26. Fine-Edelstein, J.S., Wolf, P.A., O'Leary, D.H., et al., Precursors of extracranial carotid atherosclerosis in the Framingham Study, *Neurology*, 44, 1046–1050, 1994.
27. Whisnant, J.P., Homer, D., Ingall, T.J., Baker, H.L., Jr., O'Fallon, W.M., and Wievers, D.O., Duration of cigarette smoking is the strongest predictor of severe extracranial carotid artery atherosclerosis, *Stroke*, 21, 707–714, 1990.
28. U.S. Department of Health Services, The health consequences of smoking — cardiovascular disease: a report of surgeon general, U.S. Dept of Health Services, Public Health Service, Office on Smoking and Health, Rockville, MD, 1983, DHHS publication (PHS) 84-50204.
29. Craig, W.Y., Palomaki, G.E., and Haddow, J.E., Cigarette smoking and serum lipid and lipoprotein concentrations: an analysis of published data, *Br. Med. J.*, 298, 784–788, 1989.
30. Terry, M.L., Berkowitz, H.D., and Kerstein, M.D., Tobacco: its impact on vascular disease, *Sur. Clin. North America*, 78(3), 409–429, 1998.
31. Dallongevile, J., Marecaux, N., Fruchart, J.C. et al., Cigarette smoking is associated with unhealthy patterns of nutrient intake: a meta-analysis, *J. Nutr.*, 128, 1450, 1998.

32. Henningfield, J.E., Stapleton, J.M., Benowitz, N.L. et al., Higher levels of nicotine in arterial than in venous blood after cigarette smoking, *Drug Alcohol Depend.*, 33, 23, 1993.

33. Venitt, S., Mechanisms of spontaneous human cancers, *Environ. Health Perspect.*, 104 (Suppl. 3), 633–637, 1996.

34. Blot, W.J., Alcohol and cancer, *Cancer Res.*, 52 (Suppl.), 2119s–2123s, 1992.

35. Longnecker, M.P., Alcohol consumption and risk of cancer in humans: an overview, *Alcohol*, 12, 87–96, 1995.

36. Deleyiannis, F.W., Thomas, D.B., Vaughan, T.L. et al., Alcoholism: independent predictor of survival in patients with head and neck cancer, *J. Natl. Cancer Inst.*, 88, 542–549, 1996.

37. Klygis, L.M. and Barch, D.H., The role of ethanol in esophageal carcinogenesis, in *Alcohol and Cancer*, Watson, R., Ed., CRC Press, Boca Raton, FL, 1992.

38. Seitz, H.K., Poschl, G., and Simanowski, U.A., Alcohol and cancer, *Recent Dev. Alcohol.*, 14, 67–95, 1998.

39. Peters, T.J. and Preedy, V.R., Metabolic consequences of alcohol ingestion, *Alcohol Cardiovasc. Dis.*, 216, 19–34, 1998.

40. Hoffman, D., Djordjevic, M.V., and Brunnemann, K.D., Changes in cigarette design and composition over time and how they influence the yields of smoke constituents, *J. Smoking Relat. Disord.*, 6, 9, 1995.

41. Bayer, F., Bohn, I., and Strauer, D.E., Das Kontraktionsverhalten des linen ventrikels unter nikotinexposition, *Therapiewoche*, 35, 1968, 1985.

42. Robert, D.L., Natural tobacco flavor, *Recent Adv. Tobacco Sci.*, 14, 49–81, 1988.

43. Belinsky, S.A., Deveroux, T.R., Maronpot, R.R. et al., Relation between formation of promutagenic adducts and the activation of the K-ras proto-oncogene in lung tumors in A/J mice treated with nitrosamines, *Cancer Res.*, 49, 5305, 1989.

44. Hecht, S.S. and Hoffmann, D., The relevance of tobacco-specific nitrosamines in human cancer, *Cancer Surv.*, 8, 273–294, 1989.

45. Hecht, S.S., Trushin, N., Castonguay, A. et al., A comparative tumorigenicity of DNA methylation in F344 rats by 4-(methylnitrosamino)-1-(3-pyridyl)-1-butanone and N-nitrosomethylamine, *Cancer Res.*, 46, 498–502, 1986.

46. Rodenhuis, S. and Slebos, R.J., Clinical significance of RAS activation in human lung cancer, *Cancer Res.*, 52 (Suppl. 9), 2665s–2669s, 1992.

47. Hoffman, D., Rivenson, A., and Hecht, S.S., The biological significance of tobacco-specific N-nitrosamines: smoking and adenocarcinoma, *Crit. Rev. Toxicol.*, 26, 199–211, 1996.

48. Mustonen, R., Schoket, B., and Hemminki, K., Smoking-related DNA adducts: 32P-postlabeling analysis of 7-methylguanine in human bronchial and lymphocyte DNA, *Carcinogenesis*, 14, 151, 1993.

49. Beard, M.C., Annegers, J.F., Woolner, L.B. et al., Bronchiogenic carcinoma in Olmsted County, 1935–1979, *Cancer*, 55, 2026, 1985.

50. Centers for Disease Control and Prevention, Mortality trends for selected smoking-related cancers and breast cancer — United States, 1950–1990, *MMWR*, 42, 863, 1993.

51. Muscat, J.E., Richie, J.P., Jr., Thompson, S., and Wynder, E.L., Gender differences in smoking and risk for oral cancer, *Cancer Res.*, 56, 5192, 1996.

52. Shopland, D.R., Tobacco use and its contribution to early cancer mortality with a special emphasis on cigarette smoking, *Environ. Health Perspect.*, 103, 131–141, 1995.

53. Ochsner, A. and DeBakey, M., Carcinoma of the lung, *Arch. Surg.*, 42, 209–285, 1941.
54. Henrion, D., Chillon, J.M., Capdeville-Atkinson, C. et al., Effect of chronic treatment with the calcium entry blocker, isradipine, on vascular calcium overload produced by vitamin D_3 and nicotine in rats, *J. Pharmacol. Exp. Ther.*, 260, 1–8, 1992.
55. Harley, N.H. and Cohen, B.S., Polonium-210: a questionable risk factor in smoking-related carcinogenesis, *Banbury Rep.*, 3, 93–104, 1980.
56. Mason, R.P., Walter, M.F., and Mason, P.E., Effect of oxidative stress on membrane structure: small-angle X-ray diffraction analysis, *Free Radical Biol. Med.*, 23(3), 419–425, 1997.

Index